THE ELDERCARE HANDBOOK

THE ELDERCARE HANDBOOK

Difficult Choices,
Compassionate Solutions

STELLA MORA HENRY, R.N.,
with Ann Convery

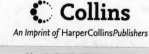
Collins

An Imprint of HarperCollinsPublishers

HarperCollins books may be purchased for educational, business, or sales promotional use. For information, please write: Special Markets Department, HarperCollins Publishers, 10 East 53rd Street, New York, NY 10022.

Designed by Emily Cavett Taff

Library of Congress Cataloging-in-Publication Data

Henry, Stella Mora.
    The eldercare handbook : difficult choices, compassionate solutions/ Stella Mora Henry with Ann Convery.—1st ed.
        p. cm.
    Includes bibliographical references and index.
    ISBN-10: 0-06-077691-9
    ISBN-13: 978-0-06-077691-6
    1. Aging parents—Care—United States. 2. Older people—Care— United States. 3 Parent and adult child—United States. I. Convery, Ann. II. Title.

HQ1063.6.H46 2006
362.61'085'40973—dc22

                                                                2005052545

    07 08 09 10 WBC/RRD 10 9 8 7 6 5 4 3

medical disclaimer

This book contains advice and information relating to health care. It is not intended to replace medical advice and should be used to supplement rather than replace regular care by your doctor. It is recommended that you seek your physician's advice before embarking on any medical program or treatment.

All efforts have been made to ensure the accuracy of the information contained in this book as of the date published. The authors and the publisher expressly disclaim responsibility for any adverse effects arising from the use or application of the information contained herein.

privacy disclaimer

The names and identifying characteristics of parents and children featured throughout this book have been changed to protect their privacy.

CONTENTS

Contents

ACKNOWLEDGMENTS

On November 11, 1969, I accepted my first position as director of nurses in a long-term-care facility. At twenty-two years of age, I had no nursing home experience; nonetheless, Mrs. Helen Hosman, the owner, "took a chance" on me. Thank you, Mrs. Hosman, for allowing me to start a journey I continue to this day. My wholehearted appreciation to the thousands of families with whom I have shared this road for allowing me to join you in your caregiving travels. To Ann Convery, I owe my heartfelt thanks for challenging me to share my experiences with others, never doubting for a moment the potential of this work. You sat hour after hour drawing this information out of me and onto paper; I am profoundly grateful. To my publicist, Anthony Mora, my appreciation for obtaining consistent media opportunities which have allowed me to shed light on eldercare issues. To Sue Brantley, thank you for your friendship and expert editing skills, which considerably enriched the book. To Harriet Bell, vice president and publisher, William Morrow Cookbooks, who had confidence in an unknown writer and allowed me to share my message, and to Toni Sciarra, my editor at Harper-Collins, who recognized my style and allowed me to communicate in my own voice—my sincere gratitude. To my sister, Pat Mora—my rock throughout this process: I am ever grateful for your continued confidence, valuable suggestions, and cheerleading skills. Christopher, thank you for understanding the importance of this project, for sharing your mother's time for the last five years, and for being a loving, helpful grandson to your beloved grandparents. You are more precious to me than you will ever know. And to my husband, Terry, without whose help I would never have been able to be the caregiver my parents needed me to be: Thank you for your love, patience, and support. You are always there for me. Finally, to Estella and Raul Mora, my treasured parents: Thank you for your unconditional love, your wisdom, and your unquestioning faith in me. I miss you daily.

INTRODUCTION:
WHAT MY FATHER TAUGHT ME

Hundreds of times I have watched hesitant families fearfully move their parents into long-term care. Yet only when I began my personal journey of relocating my own mother did I completely understand the anxiety and guilt that accompany this move.

For the past twenty-six years, my husband, Terry, and I have served as cofounders and directors of Vista del Sol Skilled Nursing and Assisted Living Facility in Los Angeles. Over the years, I have tried to anticipate families' needs to make transitions as smooth as possible. I have been guide, administrator, confidante, but none of these roles prepared me for moving my own mother.

At eighty-five, my mother walked more unsteadily as each day went by. Alzheimer's had taken her recent and long-term memories; Mom literally lived in the moment—no yesterdays to draw from, no thought of the future. She did take great pride in having reached eighty-five years of age and would remind me of it every fifteen minutes.

Moving my mother out of the apartment she had lived in for forty years was the responsible, conscientious, dutiful decision. Still, it felt strange. Until I began this personal journey, I truly thought I understood what families were going through. For years, as I kept silent watch over apprehensive daughters and sons, I would think, *They must be having a tough time arranging the move.* Little did I know. Relocating Mom opened new thresholds of guilt, fear, and anxiety. Only as I lay awake nights wondering if I'd thought of everything—would she be happy, would she miss her home, would she be angry at me—did I truly know what it meant to move a parent into long-term care.

A parade of details needed attention. After deciding the date for my mother's move, I arranged for the phone and cable TV to be connected and coordinated the furniture transfer, personalizing her room before she arrived. I chose clothing she would need, decided which pictures would have the most meaning, and arranged for Bluey, her parakeet, to be carefully transported.

As I checked off task after task, I forgot I was a registered nurse and a facility administrator. I was a daughter, an adult caregiver. Every shred of love, fear, and regret I had seen repeated in the tired, confused faces of families who had come to my office, I now felt about moving my own mother. All of us wonder if we're doing the right thing.

It Doesn't "Feel" Right

I know I made the right decision. Since a live-in daily companion could no longer address her escalating medical needs, Mom was no longer safe at home. As she grew older, the danger of a medical emergency had shadowed her days. Now, she would be safe and receive twenty-four hour professional care. Knowing that a licensed nurse would evaluate her medical needs twenty-four hours a day brought me a deep sense of relief.

Still, there were times when it just didn't feel right. The guilt we feel about moving a parent into long-term care is a normal part of the process; I see it in almost everyone who visits my office. Though I wasn't personally surprised by the guilt, it upset me all the same. These thoughts raced through my mind:

> *Maybe I can still make it work for Mom at home.*
> *Can she live with my family?*
> *She raised four of us; now we can't take care of her?*
> *Is it a good idea to uproot my mother from familiar surroundings*
> *   after forty years?*
> *What would my father say about this decision?*

Strangely, it was my father who taught me when and how to make the responsible choice for my mother.

My Father Stayed at Home

In 1990, my seventy-eight-year-old father was diagnosed with Alzheimer's. During the next three years, Dad's cognitive abilities declined rapidly, recent memory going first, followed by poor decision making. Soon, he required assistance with medication management, dressing, bathing, and toileting. Twice, he wandered away from home, frightening the whole family.

"I can take care of your dad at home," my mother pleaded with me. "Just give me a little help, and we'll be fine." The five-hour-a-day help turned into eight hours, followed by twenty-four-hour help, seven days a week. My father, a large man even though he had lost a lot of weight, required two people to transfer him in and out of a chair. He needed total nursing care.

Following his express wishes, we allowed my father to die at home. The decision was made out of emotion and guilt; at the time, I wasn't up to guiding my mother about what was really best for Dad. Although I was confidently advising families every day of my working life, when it came to facing my own family situation, I faltered. I was still my parents' child.

Most end-stage disease requires enormous medical, physical, and emotional attention. This kind of care is all-consuming, requiring medical assistance on a level too difficult to imagine until you have been there. In the next months, I logged many personal hours at my parents' apartment. Though my husband and son would have been happier if I had been home more, I went ahead and kept my promise to my dad.

I called in every IOU I had earned in the long-term care industry. The home health agency visited my father more frequently than Medicare allowed. During the last weeks of Dad's life, his skin began to break down. It didn't warrant Medicare reimbursement, but the wound nurse came anyway, as a favor to me. I built a nursing home within a home. I assembled a staff of four loving, hands-on caregivers for one-on-one twenty-four-hour care as my father lived into the end stages of Alzheimer's disease. As an RN specializing in geriatrics and long-term care, I knew it was not enough.

Dad died August 28, 1993. Through his dying process, he taught me as only he could how best to take care of my mom during her last years. Any convictions I had harbored about the sanctity of dying at home, about keeping promises out of guilt, were gone. Despite my professional expertise and contacts, Dad would have received better supervision and more comfort at a good long-term-care facility. And I would have had the time to sit with him and hold his hand.

Five years later, I again found myself making health-care decisions for a parent, but this time I felt my father's guidance. Mom needed more care than I could adequately arrange in her apartment, and the appropriate time had arrived to relocate her into a long-term-care setting. The words I have repeated to families for three decades finally came home to me: You are still your parent's advocate and champion, vitally engaged and needed more than ever. You will never relinquish the emotional care of your parent, but you can relinquish the medical care to experts.

An Emotional Roller Coaster

We are all pioneers in this strange frontier of caregiver and decision maker for parents. The learning curve is steep. Just as children do not come with instructions, neither do parents. In hundreds of interviews in my office, I have consistently heard that caregiving for an aging parent was "not supposed to happen." Mom or Dad would go quietly at the end of a long and happy life, preferably during sleep. The overwhelming role of caregiver was not something our generation saw coming, and so we find ourselves without a plan.

Much of the time, you may feel capable of meeting this caregiver challenge, able to make necessary decisions, and willing to offer emotional and financial assistance to your parents. Yet, at times, the fear, sadness, guilt, and anger can paralyze you. These disturbing feelings show up uninvited just when you thought you had them under control. Negative reactions are normal, but you must not let them deplete your strength. Whether by choice or by default you find yourself the designated caregiver, you will have signed on for the most challenging role of your life. It is an honorable position—never lose sight of that. Be prepared to make mistakes and wish you had done things differently. If you are patient and kind to yourself, both you and your parent will benefit.

Commitment Brings Peace

Walking with your parents through the final journey, whether it is months or years, can be a healing, loving time, a time for mending fences and reaching a deeper understanding. Your commitment to their care, safety, and comfort is your last and greatest gift to them. In turn, it can bring you a deep, abiding sense of peace after they are gone.

To everything there is a season. My mother lived a long and contented life at home; then, she was safely settled in the proper care center. As her primary caregiver, I was committed to providing her with compassionate care appropriate to her medical and social needs. Placing her in long-term care where I could visit with her every day was the most responsible choice I could make for her. This was the lesson my father taught me. Every time I think of his last gift to me, it brings me peace. I have written this book to share that peace with you.

1 ✎ A TIME OF CONFUSION AND UNCERTAINTY

Victor and Grace had been married sixty-two years, a lifetime, and each viewed the other as a best friend. Sitting in my office with his son, Victor felt enormous guilt talking about handing over Grace's care to someone else. With one look, I could tell he was not taking care of himself; he needed a shave and a change of shirt. While his son Tim did most of the talking, Victor alternately closed his eyes and looked at his lap. As I questioned him directly about Grace, he silently wept. I asked him how Grace spent her day. What event had made him consider long-term care?

Two months earlier, Grace was diagnosed with cancer of the kidney, and she currently required dialysis three times a week. With each procedure, she became weaker and weaker until caring for her became a formidable task. Her husband could no longer bathe and dress her or monitor her diet.

"My son says it's not fair to his mother to leave her

alone with me," Victor lamented. "I guess I just can't do it anymore."

"Victor," I gently responded, "making the responsible decision is not easy. If you allow us to become part of your caregiving team, it does not mean you will no longer care for Grace. On the contrary, it means you will begin to care for her in a different way. She will always need you to be her champion."

Where Are You Right Now?

If you are thinking about long-term care for someone, where are you in the process? Have you noticed changes in your parent, but your siblings disagree? Do you occasionally think about long-term care but feel your parent is "doing just fine" most of the time? Denial can leave you ill prepared for a future crisis.

The idea of a quick, peaceful death is a common myth. After a fulfilling life, our parents should die peacefully in their sleep. But today, the elderly live longer than ever before, and death is more likely to follow a long, weakened state or disabling illness. If talking about this brings up uncomfortable feelings, you have a lot of company. Most families who come to see me simply did not expect this to happen. They do not know what questions to ask or what to look for in a facility, but their situation is often urgent. Hospitals frequently give only twenty-four hours' notice to find a care facility.

When placing a family member in long-term care, feelings emerge that can be confusing and overwhelming. Each family brings its own dynamic to the situation. Many are truly saddened, thinking they have let their parent down. Those with no options feel trapped and angry to find themselves sitting in my office. Others may not have had a good relationship with their parent but dutifully accept the responsibility to see that needs are met. Regardless of the circumstances, I salute anyone who steps up to the plate to care for an aging parent.

Here are some stories of families who have shared the journey with me. Each one illustrates a different response to the need for long-term care.

DENIAL

Jeanne, a well-dressed, take-charge executive, came to me reluctantly. Although her seventy-nine-year-old mother, Emily, was physically strong and lived alone, she suffered from dementia. When she attempted to cross a busy boulevard against the signal, a friend stepped in and said, "Like it or not, Jeanne, you have to get involved in your mother's care. She can't live alone anymore!"

For the majority of us, denial will be the first hurdle we deal with as we step in as caregivers. As adult children, we don't always look too closely at our parents' developing needs because it's easier not to confront them. Although Jeanne had always honored her mother's choice to live independently in the comfort of her own home, Emily clearly was no longer able to manage an independent life. By not looking at her mother's situation realistically, Jeanne was neglecting the responsibility of a caregiver.

As we talked, I knew Jeanne was trying to convince me that Emily did not need help and was hoping I would confirm her assessment. Instead I said, "Jeanne, you owe your friend a thank-you. She took a risk being the bearer of news you did not want to hear."

Two months later, her mother joined us in assisted living. To Jeanne's surprise, Emily slipped easily into the new routine of meals and activities. "Except for the last few years," Jeanne admitted, "Mom has always been very social. Since my focus was on keeping her at home, I guess I gave more attention to her house than I did to her. Now that I think about it, maybe she missed being with people." Jeanne understood that denial had held her back from an earlier intervention.

ANGER

At eighty-three, Valerie needed long-term care, and her daughter Cindy was angry about it. Sitting in my office, Cindy looked tense and annoyed. Her mother had been a college dean but was now becoming forgetful, not bathing and eating regularly, and forgetting occasionally to take her medication. Cindy was convinced Valerie's lapses were intentional. "Mom had diarrhea last night," she asserted, "and I'm sure it was just a way to punish me."

Since Cindy had not had the best relationship with her mother, she was resentful of the enormous responsibility and inconvenience of taking care of her. In addition, she was angry with me and disliked being in my office as she reluctantly faced reality. And perhaps foremost, she was angry about the promise she had given Valerie years ago. "My mother made me promise never to put her in a nursing home," Cindy said.

Eventually Valerie did join us. As time went by, my staff and I became more of an advocate for Valerie than her daughter was. When Valerie's doctor ordered an antibiotic for a urinary tract infection, I notified Cindy. She was curt. "I told you, Stella," she said, "I want no aggressive care for my mother. Antibiotics are aggressive, and I don't want her to take them." Acknowledging her wishes as to caring versus curing, I nevertheless explained that this treatment was a matter of normal pain control and care, not a heroic measure. By the end of our conversation, Cindy approved the antibiotic.

Not long afterward, Valerie, who suffered from end-stage congestive heart failure, began having difficulty breathing. To ease her discomfort, oxygen was now required. Again I notified Cindy. And again, her voice was tense. "Who pays for the oxygen?" she asked impatiently. "Money is an issue, Stella."

I answered, "You will be responsible for it, Cindy, because Medicare does not reimburse for oxygen given in a nursing home."

"Does she really need it, Stella?" Cindy demanded. "Or is it only to prolong her situation?"

"Cindy," I responded, "oxygen is a comfort measure. Being short of breath is frightening, and Valerie should not experience shortness of breath or fear." After further discussion, Cindy grudgingly gave permission to order oxygen for Valerie.

During the time Valerie remained with us, Cindy was never able to resolve her anger. Although I do not know what Cindy's true feelings were, I have seen anger function in adult children as a holding pattern against sadness and grief.

SADNESS

"I had given up. I had decided I would never meet the right man. Then I met Jim," Laura began as we sat drinking coffee in my office. "When we met he was sixty, and I had just turned forty. Immediately becoming best friends, we married eight months later. For the next twenty years, we lived, as Jim described it, 'on our own private island.' I learned to sail. We traveled and saw parts of the world I had never imagined. Since Jim had three children from a previous marriage, I found myself surrounded by a good-sized family. Life was good."

Leaning across the desk, I placed a box of Kleenex in front of

Laura, who had begun to cry. "About two years ago," she said softly, "I began to notice little changes. Jim forgot things he never would have forgotten before, and he got angry with me if I drew his attention to it. This anger was new, and because being around groups of people agitated him further, I began turning down invitations."

As Laura described an elaborate system she had set up to keep Jim functioning, I felt her sadness. "How is Jim doing now?" I asked.

"After dinner last Sunday," said Laura, "Jim didn't recognize me and thought I was a stranger in the house. He asked me where Laura, his wife, had gone. As I tried to explain to him that I was Laura, he became angry and began to hit me. When he wouldn't stop, I finally had to push him back. Losing his balance, he hit his head. After I called 911, Jim was admitted to the hospital. My friends suggested I start looking into different options for when he'd be discharged," continued Laura. "I just can't believe I won't be Jim's caregiver anymore. I owe it to him."

"Laura," I said, "your caregiving does not stop the day Jim enters a nursing home. You will remain a critical source of support for Jim for the rest of his life."

"Stella, the sad thing is," said Laura, "Jim was such a wonderful man. You will never meet the person everyone loved and admired."

"Your job, Laura, will be to introduce the staff and me to the Jim that you knew. Your valuable input will help preserve his dignity and validate his individuality for us."

Joining us a week later, Jim needed assistance with bathing, dressing, and eating. Even though his communication skills were poor, when Laura entered his room, it was obvious he recognized her. His face would light up as he tried to say her name. Two weeks after Jim's arrival, Laura admitted, "I still cry at night, but I know there is no way I have the skill or stamina to properly care for my Jim anymore. In fact, I know he would back up my decision. I just wish I could stop feeling so sad about it."

"Laura," I consoled her, "the reason Jim is with us is not your lack of willingness to care for him yourself. If you had become more physically drained from caregiving than you were, you would have had nothing left to give emotionally. By making the long-term-care decision, you have entered into a partnership with us to provide the physical care that you can no longer adequately provide. But no one will be able to replace the love and affection you give Jim. You are his connection between his old home and his new home."

GRIEF

Fay, ninety-eight, had been with us for four years and was dying of cancer. At eighty, her son Stan had been his mother's caregiver for twenty years. "Mom has always been fragile, in need of my care," said Stan. "Relocating her into assisted living was the most difficult decision I've ever made. I felt as though I were giving up a part of myself." Every morning at ten and again every afternoon around five, Stan visited his mother, but lately he was having a hard time dealing with his mother's mortality. In the past, Stan had always stopped in to chat with me after he saw his mother. As Fay weakened, Stan's visits with me became less frequent. At the same time, he became unrealistically demanding with the staff, even instructing that the nurses get Fay in and out of bed every half hour. In her condition, this would have been much too hard on Fay. When told that Fay was only eating 20 percent of her lunch, Stan became upset. He tried feeding her himself, but she would not eat for him, either. Frequently, as he entered his mother's room, he became teary and emotional. During one of his visits, I asked him to come back to my office. "Stan," I said, "you have been her son for eighty years. Whether you are fifty or eighty, the loss of your mother will bring enormous grief."

"I know, Stella, I know. I lost my father thirty years ago, and even though I'm eighty now, I'm having a hard time letting go of my mother. It's almost like I'm not sure who I'll be when she's gone."

No matter how old we are, parents give us a sense of place in the social order. Even if you no longer go to them for advice, it is a secure feeling just knowing that you have parents. The loss of the second parent is a transition for which few of us are prepared; we find ourselves not only orphaned but facing our own mortality.

GUILT

"I knew I was in trouble," Debby said, "when my mom, Anita, got up from the sofa and it was stained with urine." Diagnosed four years ago with Parkinson's and dementia, Anita had managed fairly well for a while. "But by the time Mom came to live with us last year," Debby continued, "she was losing weight, not changing her clothes, and forgetting to take medication. In just the last two weeks, Mom has taken a sudden spiral downward. Now that incontinence is an issue, she is taking up a lot more of my time, and I have a two-year-old daughter who's competing for my attention. To complicate matters, Mom has had a couple of falls and just yesterday fractured two ribs. Now she's getting confused at night; when she walked into our bedroom at three A.M. by mistake, I actually yelled at her. Although my husband loves my mom and has been a real trooper this last year, his primary concerns are my little girl and me. He told me, 'You're a nervous wreck. Things have to change.' How do I tell

Mom she needs more care than we can give her at home? I feel so much guilt over this decision!"

"Debby," I said, "as we become caregivers to our aging parents, we will always experience some guilt. Falling, incontinence, and confusion at night are all signs that your mother needs more care. At this point in your life, are you able to provide her with all the care she needs? That is the question you have to answer. As caregivers, we find ourselves attempting to solve all of our children's problems and all our parents' problems as well. Most of us can't do it. But we can be our parents' advocate, finding a quality long-term-care facility when it's needed, and we can continue to be actively involved in their health care."

The following day, Anita joined us. The relocation phase for Anita took about two weeks. Initially, she would not attend activities and her appetite was poor. Even her granddaughter could not cheer her up. As her family visited daily, the staff continued to encourage Anita to attend activities and special events. Throughout the day, Precious, our facility dog, visited Anita. One morning, Anita unexpectedly said, "Okay, little doggie, you can be on the bed with me." Precious hopped up. That was the beginning of Anita's transition to her new environment. Soon, she began to ask for Precious after breakfast, and the little dog would ride in the wheelchair with her to activities. Family visits became less strained and more meaningful.

"I think," said Debby tearfully, "when Mom has a clear day, she knows that I can't care for her anymore. I hope she does."

The role conflict Debby was experiencing is common among middle-aged daughters and daughters-in-law who find themselves parent, spouse, and caregiver in addition to housekeeper and employee. Debby's loyalty to her mother was real. Yet her concern for her family was equally real. Guilt, or fear of guilt, can cloud one's ability to make responsible decisions. But with the help of her husband and with clear, honest communication, they were able to confront the situation and bring it to a resolution that worked for everyone.

As a caregiver, you will always feel guilt to some degree. But once you acknowledge you can't do everything for everybody, guilt loses some of its power.

Assuming the Caregiver's Role

I hope the stories of others who have made this journey will help you as you begin the difficult, delicate road to caring for your aging loved one. There are classes on how to care for newborns, toddlers, and preteens, but classes on caring for aging parents are few and far between—there are no real guidelines. Each family will have different needs, circumstances, and interpersonal dynamics.

Knowing how long to allow a parent in transition to make her own decisions is a tough call. At what point is it necessary to step in? When Jeanne described her mother's precarious walk across the boulevard, I said to her, "Just as you cannot leave a child home alone, you cannot leave parents who are no longer able to make safe decisions." They need safe boundaries.

Jeanne felt strongly that her mother would want to maintain her independence, yet allowing Emily to live alone when she could not sense danger crossing a busy street would have been irresponsible. As those of us who have gone through it can confirm, becoming your parents' decision maker is a time of awakening. In the past, we looked to them for advice, opinions, assistance, and protection; now we return the favor. While it is not an easy role to slip into, it is a gift we give our parents: good, appropriate care for the remainder of their lives, whether at home or in a quality facility.

If You Can't Step in as a Caregiver

Perhaps your parents are not ready to allow you to step in and make decisions with them. If they won't relinquish car keys or accept help at home, they may be unwilling even to consider the notion of long-term care. Remember that if your parent is mentally alert, she should make her own decisions, whether you agree or not. However, if your parent is placing herself in imminent danger, or if her health is seriously threatened, you do have the responsibility to become involved. At least have a backup plan in place to avoid finding yourself in a crisis with nowhere to go. Here is how you can start:

1. Educate yourself about local agencies that provide home-care services which may include everything from shopping and cooking assistance to twenty-four-hour care. Also inquire at the local senior center for possible future part-time help. In many communities, people offer their services by the hour to do errands, cook, or just sit with older adults. Investigate Meals on Wheels.

2. Be sure your parents have both signed a durable power of attorney for health care (DPA; called advance health care directive in California) and a durable power of attorney for finances. These documents appoint an agent—usually a trusted family member or friend—to act in your parents' place to make health-care and financial decisions in the event they are unable to do so themselves.

3. Familiarize yourself now with long-term-care options such as assisted living and nursing home facilities in your neighborhood. (See Chapter 11 for different levels of long-term care.)

4. If you are a long-distance caregiver, enlist the help of a friendly neighbor to keep an eye on your parents and to keep you posted regarding behavior changes. Or, investigate the services of a geriatric-care manager (see Chapter 12) in your parents' area.

Unfortunately, you may have to wait for the inevitable car accident, fall, or medical crisis before you are able to step in and help your parents. If a call comes from the emergency room, and one of your parents has broken a hip or suffered a stroke, you won't have much time to think about the next level of care; frequently hospitals will not notify you of a discharge decision until there is only twenty-four hours to find a facility. In a crisis, it is difficult to make a major decision to best suit your parent.

Seventeen Hours to Find a Nursing Home

On a Tuesday morning, Betsy sat in my office, anxious, angry, and frightened. Ever since Betsy's mother died, her eighty-nine-year-old father, Larry, had lived alone and seemed self-sufficient. However, when Betsy visited him that Friday afternoon, he was disoriented, hadn't changed his clothes for a few days, and felt hot to the touch. "The ER doctor told me that along with a temperature of 103.2, Dad had a severe urinary tract infection," said Betsy. That night, Larry was admitted to the hospital. At six-thirty Monday night, the hospital discharge planner informed Betsy that Larry had to leave the hospital by the next morning and would need a nursing home. "How," she asked the discharge planner, "am I going to find a nursing home by tomorrow morning, if I only have tonight to see them?"

Betsy continued, "I went home, and began calling anyone I could think of—friends, relatives—to see if they knew of a facility. Finally, I reached my rabbi, who gave me your name. Do you have room for my dad?"

Regrettably, I had to reply, "I'm so sorry, Betsy, I won't have a bed until next week. Let me make some calls for you and see if there's a bed in a facility I can recommend." The majority of nursing home admissions from the hospital are made under this type of pressure.

Have a Plan

Armed with knowledge and a plan, you will have more choice and more control. A plan stabilizes a crisis; it replaces confusion with assurance. As your parents enter their eighties or nineties, they will need guidance and support. Although you may feel you can and must do everything for them, this may be an unrealistic expectation, a prescription for heartbreak which can lead to denial, anger, sadness, grief, and guilt. With a flexible plan in place, these ever-present feelings lose some of their power. While there are no perfect answers, preparation, communication, and a realistic assessment of your parent's situation will lead to sound decisions.

"**S**ince Dad died two years ago, Mom has done amazingly well," Elizabeth told me. "Her house isn't as clean as it used to be, but it's still pretty neat. I can't really explain why I worry about her being alone." As I questioned Elizabeth about her eighty-year-old mother's housekeeping, she interrupted me and said, "Stella, to answer you, I'd have to snoop around like a detective whenever I visit Mom."

"That's not a bad analogy," I replied. "In a sense, we do need to become detectives to help our parents continue to live safely. There may be faint warnings of physical or cognitive disabilities to come. These 'red flags' alert you when a parent begins to need more care. It might mean extra help around the house, more medical attention, or a review of medications."

"To tell the truth," continued Elizabeth, "I'm not sure she's keeping track of her finances, and I'm worried about what she's eating."

"Nobody knows your mother as well as you do," I said. "If you think there might be problems, there probably are. The sooner you identify red flags, the sooner you can begin to shape a plan for the future before a serious event occurs."

Assessing lifestyle changes is a highly personal journey for you and your parents, and there are no hard-and-fast rules. Although you may be uncomfortable entering your parents' home knowing you are there to check up on them, it may be a valuable service. To help assess how well your parents are doing, I have compiled a list of ten common red flags, starting with personal care.

I. Personal Care

- Are there buttons missing from your parent's clothing?
- Is your parent's clothing unkempt or unclean?
- Does she wear the same clothes day after day?
- Is there body odor?
- Does it look as if your parent is not brushing her teeth regularly?
- Has your mother stopped caring about her hair and makeup?
- Has your father stopped shaving and getting regular trims?

Chris and Lili. Chris came to see me about his ninety-two-year-old mother, Lili, who lived alone in Beverly Hills. A physician, Chris felt he had covered all of Lili's needs by carefully putting many support systems in place for her. To him, Lili seemed alert. She had always been a social, elegant woman who dressed beautifully and loved parties. She seemed to be doing fine on her own.

During a visit to his mother, however, he noticed that she now wore the same housedress every time he saw her. He also noticed a musty odor in the house. It dawned on him that Lili probably had not been bathing. "I think she was pouring on the perfume whenever I came to visit," he told me later. Since the odor was a subtle change in his mother's behavior, he did not consider it important. By the time Lili joined us, her personal hygiene needed immediate intervention. The mere mention of a bath made her nervous and fearful.

Bathing can be a frightening experience for the elderly. It takes considerable coordination and organization, and your parent may not be up to the task. Simply adjusting the hot and cold water controls in the shower can get confusing. It may also be difficult for older people to maintain their balance as they step in and out of the bathtub. In Lili's case, she didn't want to bathe because she was afraid of falling. In grabbing the sliding bathtub door to steady herself, she could have lost her footing and fractured her hip—a common accident among the elderly.

As small changes take place, you can lose a lot of valuable time before noticing a parent's true condition. If your mother has always worn attractive shoes that matched her outfits, but is now wearing old slippers, this is a significant change. On the other hand, switching from comfortable old tennis shoes to comfortable old slippers might not be significant.

II. Housekeeping

- Are the appliances and silverware sticky?
- Have any utilities been turned off because bills have not been paid?
- Is the refrigerator in need of a thorough cleaning?
- Is there an accumulation of garbage or spoiled food?
- Are the carpets stained?

- Are the bedsheets soiled?
- Is your parent reluctant to accept outside help?

Stewart and Amy. Stewart had been watching over his eighty-eight-year-old mother, Amy, for the past two years. "I never really worried about her," Stewart said. "I took her grocery shopping, and she did the rest. Last week when I opened her refrigerator, there was more food than usual, and it didn't smell good. Seeing the look on my face, Mom urged me out the door, saying, 'Let's go. I'll tidy that up when I get back.' The following week when I checked the refrigerator situation, what I found scared me. The foul odor had intensified. Food needed to be thrown out, and the refrigerator needed a good scrubbing. Heck, the entire kitchen needed attention. That was the moment it hit me—Mom needed help."

It is difficult to accept that your parent is no longer able to care for himself. As one man shared with me, "Stella, my father is a retired superior court judge. Stepping into his life to help or intervene is hard to imagine." Is your parent aware he needs help, or is he unaware? Either way, a comprehensive medical evaluation will determine if the cause is physical or cognitive. Could depression be a factor? A family physician *with experience in caring for the elderly* can provide helpful insights.

III. Meals and Appetite

- Is the refrigerator nearly empty?
- Is the food you brought three or four days ago still uneaten?
- Is your parent relying solely on TV dinners?
- Does he have trouble chewing because of ill-fitting dentures?
- Has there been noticeable weight gain or loss?

"Following my dad's death," said Vincent, "my mother stopped preparing dinner, something she had done every night at six o'clock for fifty-two years. Now it looks like she's losing weight. When I asked her about her diet, she said, 'If there's no one to enjoy the meal with, it's not worth cooking.'"

The need for assistance in buying and preparing food may begin very subtly. Meals are a social time for most of us. If your parent is living alone and has lost a spouse or good friend, his appetite may diminish. Perhaps your parent can't see clearly enough to read cooking instructions, or maybe arthritis prevents her from handling pots and pans and silverware. Dental problems can make eating difficult or painful. In addition, certain medications affect appetite while others cause the mouth to be uncomfortably dry.

IV. Memory

- Does your parent call you at work for no apparent reason?
- Are you getting phone calls from your parent in the middle of the night?
- Does your parent call you with the same question several times a day?
- Is your parent unable to remember his previous calls?
- Is your parent's phone bill higher than usual?

"Mom started calling me every night to let me know she was going to bed," said Roy of his eighty-seven-year-old parent. "Five minutes later, she would call again, and repeat the same loving message. By the fourth call, I felt like unplugging the phone."

If your parent calls frequently asking trivial questions about dinner or the weather, this may indicate a need for attention or a lack of stimulation. But watch for a pattern of repetition; if she calls four or five times a day with the same question, test the waters by saying, "Mom, have you already called me today about this?" This gentle question will not offend or frighten your parent, but will help you assess her situation. When she honestly cannot remember she has already called, you will know this is a behavior change that needs to be addressed.

It doesn't matter how good-natured you are, when that same phone call with the same question keeps coming over and over, there will be a day when you lose patience. Try to remember that your parent is responding to thoughts that are perfectly logical to her and that she will have no idea why you are upset. To her it's a brand-new call. If you do lose your temper, remember that every other adult caregiver has done this, and probably more than once. You may feel the impulse to call your parent back to apologize. However, if your parent has no recollection of your anger, an apology might only confuse her. If her memory lapses continue, contact her physician and request a cognitive assessment. (For more about cognitive assessments, see Chapter 7: "My Mother Doesn't Have Alzheimer's, But…")

V. Communication

- Does your parent have difficulty following directions?
- Is she confused by the TV remote or the portable phone?
- Does he frequently search for the right word during conversation?

Nathalie and Her Mom. Nathalie, a petite, elegant woman in her late sixties, leaned over the desk as she described her mother to me. "My mother is extraordinarily intelligent," she asserted. "She taught at the college level for twenty years and speaks three languages, so I can't understand what the problem is. I tried to teach her how to put a cassette in a tape recorder. I said to her, 'Mom! Stick the tape in the slot and put the lid down! Is that so hard?' My brother Jack has given up on her. He told me, 'Nathalie, don't argue with her. You know what the doctor said about her memory.' And I said, 'I will not patronize my mother. I'm not going to talk down to her.' But I just can't get her to use that tape recorder. Every time I try to help her, she gets more upset and confused. Sometimes she can't remember a word, or she says the wrong word. I tell her, 'Mom, I cannot understand you; you have to say it again.' I won't let her give in to this!"

"Nathalie," I said gently, "You mom's memory isn't what it used to be. Think of her mind as a tall building with all the lights on. A light goes out on the top floor, and another light goes out on the fifth floor, and so on. Eventually, the whole building will go dark. Nathalie, your mother can't keep up with you anymore."

She looked at me and began to cry softly. "I'm losing her, aren't I?" she said.

As adult children, we do not want to accept that our parents cannot follow directions, or that they get easily confused and anxious. It scares us for our own sake as well as for theirs. Diminished communication is a warning sign that your parent is beginning to lose cognitive abilities. If you frequently find yourself exasperated at your parent's inability to follow a conversation, it is time for an assessment by a physician well versed in cognitive disorders.

VI. Mobility

- Does your parent have difficulty going up and down stairs?

- Does your parent have the strength to get out of a soft chair by herself?
- Is your parent's balance unsteady after rising from a sitting position?
- Can your parent get in and out of a car without assistance?

If you have noticed your parent's movements are more slow, stiff, and unsteady, it may be time for an assessment by his physician; in fact, an evaluation by a physical therapist might be in order. Ben told me, "I knew Dad was having problems when he grabbed his walker to pull himself out of the car and both he and the walker toppled backward." Fortunately, since an elder's physical decline is often due to inactivity, mobility is one area that can be improved through exercise. Exercise is also known to reduce arthritis pain, improve sleeping habits, and increase mobility and energy levels. Consult your parent's physician for an appropriate and safe exercise program.

VII. Depression: Losing Interest in Life

- Was your mother a passionate reader who has now lost interest in books?
- Was your father an avid sports fan who no longer watches games on TV?
- Has your mother abandoned her knitting needles?
- Has your parent lost interest in food?
- Is your parent turning down invitations she once looked forward to?
- Is your parent becoming moody, anxious, or angry for no apparent reason?

Of course, altered behavior can have physical causes. Your mother may not be able to read small print anymore. Your father may have stopped watching TV because he can't hear. Your mother may not knit because of arthritis. Or all of the above could be caused by depression.

Bret and Karen. At eighty-seven, Bret lived alone after his wife died. His daughter Karen said her father had always been a very social man, and it saddened her to see him withdrawing. Whereas he used to count the days until his grandchildren's visits, now he showed little interest in seeing them. He began to lose weight. His depression deepened. When Karen took him to UCLA Neuropsychiatric Institute, he was admitted for clinical depression. After he was discharged, Bret joined us in assisted living. It took him about a week to join our activities and really interact with the group. We found that he loves to dance, and he has become quite the romantic hero with the ladies. Given the title Official Greeter, Bret goes out of his way to help new residents with their first few days of relocation. Residents who have led highly social lives frequently benefit from the stimulation they receive in community living.

People over sixty-five cope with an increasing number of losses—death of loved ones, financial problems, feelings of powerlessness, physical disabilities, chronic pain, social isolation, and diminished memory. Any one of these can cause depression; cumulatively, they can be devastating.

A silent predator, depression not only damages quality of life, but also takes a toll on physical health. Symptoms may include insomnia, fatigue, loss of appetite, and changes in daily activities. But depression should not be considered a normal part of aging; it is treatable and needs to be evaluated just as you would a medical illness.

VIII. Medication

- Do your parent's medications have expired dates?
- Are the bottles too full considering when the prescriptions were purchased?
- Are the bottles too empty; has she taken too much?
- Are medications from multiple pharmacies?
- Is there an excessive number of over-the-counter medications, such as aspirin, cough syrups, or antacids?

My Mom and I. At age eighty-two, my mother prided herself on being able not only to recite all thirteen of her medications, but also to tell you the purpose of each drug. Each Sunday for the past several weeks, I had stopped by to see Mom in the early afternoon. Typically, I would find her ritually preparing her medications for the coming week. Thirteen bottles of medication would be neatly lined up in a row as she diligently poured each medication into her seven-day organizer. This particular afternoon, I heard my mother mutter to herself, "What have I done now?" Peeking into the dining room, I saw Mom staring at the medication bottles, looking very puzzled. "Mom," I said, "let me lend you a hand today, so we can sit and visit. I'll take the container, and you hand me the pills." Looking down, I found two of the same pills in Monday's slot and none in Tuesday's or Wednesday's. How long had there been a problem? It was my first red flag that my mother had entered a stage in her life where she needed guidance and support.

Due to the large number of pills elderly people take every day, medications are a serious area of concern. If your parent is taking ten different drugs a day, which is not uncommon, and if the medication schedule varies for each pill, keeping track can become a real headache. If you have not already done so, make a list of your parent's current medications. Tactfully checking your parent's medication bottles, look at the dates when they were filled, and figure how many pills should still be in the bottles. Keep in mind that our parents may see three to four different specialists, each of whom prescribes medications within his own specialty. Often, medications contraindicate one another as various physicians fail to look at the whole medical regime.

Georgia. Georgia, eighty-seven, lived alone. Following an acute episode of irregular heartbeat, she was given blood thinner medication for stroke prevention as well as prednisone for severe bronchitis. Three weeks later, her doctor prescribed a baby aspirin, which was meant to replace the blood thinner. Instead, Georgia took both the aspirin and the blood thinner. All three medications she was taking could cause bleeding. During her last visit to the doctor, Georgia's lab work showed she was anemic. As a result, she was placed on a daily dose of iron, which in turn caused a constipation problem. No one thought to look at the whole picture. On the day of her admission to assisted living, we asked the doctor for lab work to assess Georgia's blood levels. Our lab reported a hemoglobin level so abnormal that Georgia required immediate hospitalization and two units of blood. Not surprisingly, each of the three medications Georgia had been taking had ordered by a different specialist. With her medications reevaluated, she returned to assisted living, taking only baby aspirin.

According to the California Pharmacists Association, as many as one hundred thousand Americans die from adverse drug reactions every year. Millions more are injured. Ideally, all your parent's medications should be filled at one pharmacy. Ask a trusted pharmacist to review your parent's current medications. Be sure to include all over-the-counter drugs she is currently taking, since they can interact with prescription drugs. The pharmacist will let you know if there are any contraindications you should address with the doctor.

IX. Finances

- Has your parent paid the gas bill twice?
- Are there piles of unopened mail?
- Are there final-notice letters from collection agencies?
- Is your parent's bank account overdrawn?
- Are there frequent unexplained transfers from savings to checking?

Suzette and Her Dad. "My dad is an eighty-four-year-old retired psychologist who worked in counseling for thirty-two years," began Suzette, an attractive redhead in her sixties. "In retirement, he made ends meet with Social Security and some investments he had made. Dad's entertainment was going out to dinner on Tuesdays, Thursdays, and Saturdays with friends. About a year ago, I noticed he was eating at home on Tuesdays and Thursdays. The following week, I invited Dad to join my husband and me for dinner. Driving home after we dropped him off, my husband remarked to me, 'Did you see all the thank-yous from different charities on your dad's desk? There had to be at least ten.' Stella, I had to bring this up with Dad, but I wasn't sure how to go about it."

"Gathering financial information is tricky," I told Suzette. "Since finances are a private area, you may appear to be prying with the simplest question, and your dad may feel threatened or uncomfortable."

"That's for sure!" Suzette exclaimed. "My questions about his financial statements did not go over well. But the thank-you notes were still on the dining room table and there was over seven hundred dollars in donations. Also, his checkbook hadn't been balanced in eight months. To make a long story short, Dad finally did go over his finances with me. Not only was he skipping dinners, but he was also cutting some of his medications because he couldn't afford them! I'm not sure Dad even remembered giving to all those organizations. After I took over his finances, he could afford all his medications and his beloved dinners again."

Because personal finance is as closely tied to your parent's sense of independence as driving is, financial issues are among the most difficult to discuss. Don't be surprised if your parent is uncomfortable sharing his financial status, but try to have a discussion *before* there is a need for intervention, so if a problem arises, you can effectively step in.

How do you begin the conversation? You could try a version of the following: "Dad, I'm worried I won't be able to help you with your banking if you ever have a medical emergency. When Marcy's father had a stroke, she had no idea of his financial situation, and now he is unable to tell her. Since she can't access his accounts, Marcy is struggling to pay all his household and medical bills." Or, you could say, "Mom, I'm starting a retirement plan that I hope will cover my living expenses. How did you plan your retirement? Is it working?"

If your parent is alert and does not feel comfortable divulging financial information to you or anyone else in the family, suggest he speak with a trusted attorney or financial planner.

X. Driving

- Has your father incurred an increasing number of traffic violations?
- Has he been involved in a number of small accidents?
- Are there unexplained dents or scrapes on the car?

- Does your mother drive at an unsafe speed, too slow or too fast?
- Do you feel it is necessary to call to see if your parents ar-rived home safely?
- Does your parent ever get lost while driving?
- Would you ride with your parent?
- Would you let your children ride with your parent?

William, Gert, and Matthew. William, eighty-six, visited his wife, Gert, twice a day at the nursing home. Matthew, their only child, had a growing concern about his dad's driving ability. When Gert still lived at home, William had allowed a driver to take them to Gert's dialysis treatments. But now that Gert was in a nursing home, he stated adamantly, "I don't need a driver!"

Their son lobbied to have a caregiver drive his father twice a day for visits. "He has no business driving," said Matthew. "He doesn't always look both ways, and he switches lanes without signaling."

Two weeks later Matthew called me, anxious and frightened. "Stella, I just got a call. Dad's been in an accident. He's in the emer-gency room. I'm on my way there now." William had hit an eigh-teen-year-old girl who suffered a fractured wrist and lacerations over one eye, requiring stitches. William himself had fractured four ribs and his pelvis. Close to tears, Matthew admitted to me, "I knew I should have taken those keys away, but Dad put up such a fuss, it was easier to let the situation slide. Now I feel responsible for Dad and that poor girl."

Many families have to wait for unexplained dents or minor acci-dents before broaching the subject of surrendering car keys. Re-member: Loss of driving privileges equals loss of independence in our society, especially for men. If you are the bearer of the bad news, don't be surprised if resentment descends on you full force. If your parent is mentally alert and able to make his own decisions, there will be a limit to the intervention you can offer. Having said that, if his driving is placing him and others in clear and imminent danger, you must act. Find a person to whom your parent will listen. It may be a grandchild who says, "Papa, I'm worried about your driving," or it might be your family physician. Chances are, your parent will value the doctor's recommendation more than yours.

The Time to Start Is Now

Does your father have problems with his personal hygiene because he doesn't notice, because he doesn't care, or because it's too hard to keep up? Could his condition be a combination of all three? As his caregiver, you must make it your job to figure it out. If personal hygiene is not the first red flag, it may be banking activities and complicated financial problems that need your attention. Perhaps housekeeping has become an issue, or your mother has lost the ability to communicate how she spent her day. Start observing your parent now. Pay attention to the red flags, and create a plan. If your parent can be involved in the planning, it not only allows him to retain his role as decision maker for the remainder of his life as you carry out his financial, medical, and end-of-life wishes, but it also simplifies your role as caregiver.

CHECKLIST:
Red Flags to Watch For

1. **Personal Care**: Deteriorated personal hygiene, uncombed hair, soiled clothing, mismatched clothing, difficulty getting in and out of tub or shower without assistance, infrequent bathing, incontinence.

2. **Housekeeping**: Accumulation of garbage or spoiled food, stained carpets, piles of dirty laundry, unclean silverware, sticky kitchen counter, reluctance to accept help.

3. **Meals and Appetite**: Difficulty preparing meals, decreased appetite, noticeable weight loss or gain, stale food, empty refrigerator.

4. **Memory**: Forgetting appointments and names, repeating stories in conversation, regularly losing or misplacing objects, loss of recent memory, repeated phone calls for the same reason, forgetting how to use the telephone.

5. **Communication**: Difficulty finding specific words, increasingly illegible handwriting, difficulty learning or retaining new information.

6. **Mobility**: Slower pace when walking, difficulty climbing stairs, unsteady gait, frequent falls, balance problems.

7. **Depression**: Unexplainable anxiety or irritability, decreased interest in family or friends, avoidance of previously enjoyed activities.

8. **Medication**: Frequently missed daily medications, difficulty recalling if medication was taken, overuse of medications, untimely reordering of medications.

9. **Finances**: Unopened mail, unpaid bills or bills paid twice, unbalanced or overdrawn checkbook, unexplained credit card charges, frequent transfers from savings into checking accounts, threatening letters from collection agencies.

10. **Driving**: Unsafe driving speed, difficulty negotiating turns, unexplained dents or scrapes, increased traffic violations, difficulty parking.

3 ✍ DENIAL

enial is an equal opportunity phenomenon. Crossing educational and income barriers, it affects 95
percent of families who come to my office. Even physicians and psychiatrists are unable to be objective regarding their parents' needs. It amazes me how denial
can cause a loving family to overlook the many warning
signs. Interestingly, denial is the first step most of us experience in caregiving. By the time you find yourself
making excuses for your parents' forgetfulness or behavior, you have already started caregiving, whether you
realize it or not.

As a defense mechanism, denial can provide two
things: (1) time to absorb changes you are not ready to
cope with, and (2) a chance to regroup for the tasks
ahead. Not until I became primary caregiver for my
own parents could I begin to understand the process.
Because changes in our parents' appearance and behavior can be so easily rationalized, appropriate assistance

is often delayed two or three years. When seniors are forgetful, a grown son or daughter can say, "Mom's always been like this," or "It's not the first time she's gotten information mixed up." These responses keep us in an emotionally safe cocoon where, if no problem exists, everything must be okay. None of us likes the changes in our parents' lives, yet time will not stand still. At some point, we will no longer be able to pretend all is well.

The Family in Denial

Seeing denial in my own family was an awakening experience. When the graduation invitation for my parents' youngest granddaughter arrived from Texas, we booked our flights to El Paso. As they had several times over the past fifteen years, Mom and Dad stayed with my sister Cecilia. One afternoon I observed my dad standing in her hallway, looking perplexed. "What's up, Dad?" I asked jokingly.

He stared at me and asked, "Where am I, Stella?"

He wasn't joking. He was lost. "You're visiting Cecilia," I answered. "Your bedroom is behind you." Looking back, he saw two doors, one to the bedroom, the other to a closet. He asked me which door he should go to. Directing him to the bedroom, I thought, That's strange, and tried to forget the incident. Denial.

A few hours later, I spoke to my sisters Pat and Cecilia. "Something odd happened," I told them. "Dad got lost in your house, Cecilia. Now that I think about it, there have been small changes taking place in his behavior."

"Oh, Stella," they both answered too quickly, "you worry too much about Dad! You always have. He looks and acts fine. Just last night we reminisced about the good old days and he was right on target."

Telling me not to worry, they agreed to keep an eye on Dad. I was only too happy to take their advice. "They're probably right," I rationalized, "Dad's fine." More denial.

When we returned to Los Angeles, things went well for two months. Then, one day, Mom called. Dad had been working on his coin collection when she noticed he was mismarking them. "I know what he paid for those coins," she said, "and he's giving them away at these prices."

"Do you want me to talk to him about it?" I asked.

"Yes, honey, please come over tomorrow," said Mom. But the following morning, she told me to forget about it; things were okay.

Again, I was happy to agree, thinking, Who would know better than Mom? He's fine. Still more denial? Several other incidents had to take place before it was clear I could not ignore his behavior any longer. I began calling my mother every day and dropping by at least three times a week to see how Dad was doing. As my father began to exhibit early-stage dementia, I was taking the first small steps on a four-year journey caring for him.

Caring for aging parents makes us face facts. We must deal not only with the reality of their frailties, but with our own as well. Not expecting to live this long, most of our parents have no long-term health plan. As it falls to us to create a plan for their long-term needs, it dawns on us that we will eventually have to create one for ourselves; thus, we begin to face our own mortality.

The Out-of-Town Sibling in Denial

In my experience, denial is prevalent in siblings who live away from the parent, whereas the day-to-day caregiver in the thick of the situation sees the subtle changes taking place. When observations are shared with the family, they are frequently not taken seriously.

One morning, Bonnie, a city comptroller, was waiting anxiously in my office when I arrived. "I know I don't have an appointment," she began, "but I was wondering if you could give me some information about your facility." Bonnie had come to see me about her eighty-one-year-old mother, Esther. "Mom lives alone," she went on, "and my sister Sarah who lives out of state thinks Mom leads an independent life. However, she has no idea the effort it takes on my part to keep Mom 'independent.' Last week, I wrote to her that Mom has not been herself, that she's wandering around her own house appearing to be lost. Writing back, my sister responded, 'You're tired and probably overreacting. When I saw Mom last month, she looked great.'"

"Stella," said Bonnie, "It's so frustrating. Whenever Sarah visits, Mom looks great because I make it my business to make her look great. If Sarah would stick around for three weeks, she would see how Mom really is."

"What does your mother need that Sarah doesn't see?" I asked Bonnie.

"If Sarah and I traded places for three weeks, she'd have to go shopping and buy only certain brand names, or Mom won't use them. She'd have to fill the gas tank, and check the car for new dents. She'd have to pay the bills, balance the checkbook, and order all Mom's medicines. And that's just the beginning. Mom is a full-time job."

Resentment can creep into the best of sibling relationships because the hands-on caregiver is acutely aware of the difference between a special visit and day-to-day, hour-by-hour care. The hands-on caregiver may feel isolated by the lack of understanding and support from siblings. Even brothers and sisters who are good friends may have to reassess their relationship as a new family dynamic begins.

If you are a secondary or distance caregiver, start by asking how you can help. Perhaps you can offer more financial assistance, or sit in for the main caregiver so she can have an afternoon off or a weekend away. Ask regularly if there is some shopping you can do, such as pajamas, underwear, groceries, or perfume. Families tend to think, If she needed help, she would ask for it. Not necessarily. Primary caregivers traditionally are not good at asking for help.

Walk a Mile in Your Sister's Shoes

Sitting across from me late one Thursday afternoon, Rebecca, Louise, and Robert each appeared concerned. "Mom is eighty-nine," began Rebecca, the primary caregiver. "She tries hard and she's so sweet and kind, but I just can't take care of her at home anymore. I've told Robert and Louise how I feel."

Louise interrupted, "Rebecca, I live only six hours away. We shouldn't even be talking about assisted living. The three of us can divide the responsibility. It can't be that difficult. If Mom raised the three of us, we ought to be able to take care of her. She loves to talk about the past, and is a perfect hostess when I visit."

"Louise," said Robert, "you visit for a few hours twice a month. Mom is the perfect hostess because Rebecca gets her all dressed up, cleans her house, and prepares the food she gives you. You and Mom just sit and talk. I help out one or two times a week, and by the time I leave, I'm exhausted."

"Louise," I interceded, "how would you feel about taking your mom to your home over the weekend? That would give Rebecca a needed break and help you understand your mom's needs."

"If that will keep Mom independent," Louise quickly responded, "I'll do it."

The experience proved to be an eye-opener. Louise picked her mother up Friday afternoon; by Saturday night, she brought her mother right back to Rebecca's.

"Mother looked so good," Louise later shared with me, "that I just didn't get it. About an hour after we got to my house, Mom began looking for Rebecca. No matter how many times I explained to her where Rebecca was, she just kept asking the same question over and over. This went on all day. When a friend invited us to dinner, we were there less than an hour when Mom insisted she had to get home before it started raining, although there was no rain predicted. She was so frightened, I couldn't calm her down. All I could do was bring her back to Rebecca. Now I know she can't stay at home." A week later, their mom joined us in assisted living.

Clear communication is the heart of a good care system. The main players need to sit down and deal with health, financial, and end-of-life issues. Since this is difficult to do by phone or e-mail, families should make an effort to have a face-to-face meeting. Use the meeting plan outlined in Chapter 5, Redefining Sibling Roles, to get you started. A plan enables everyone to know in advance what the options are and helps families deal with complex emotions and the inevitable denial.

Dementia Can Reinforce Denial

One of the confusing aspects about dementia is that your parent can continue to display social graces that can stay intact well into the second stage, thus reinforcing the family's denial. In fact, denial of cognitive disability can be so strong it reawakens old sibling rivalries. For example, if the primary caregiver says, "Dad's limping," siblings are concerned and may ask how they can help, or suggest he be taken to a doctor. However, if she says, "Dad's been forgetting things like shaving and taking his medicine," siblings may bristle at the information and challenge it.

Depending on the parent's cognitive abilities, a secondary caregiver may not get a true picture of the situation because brief visits don't reflect day-to-day reality. So, if you are a secondary caregiver, realize that your visits may be carefully orchestrated for your benefit and may be reinforcing your denial.

The Primary Caregiver in Denial

In a consultation with me about his family, Bill, a retired accountant, explained, "My sister Mary is a seventy-two-year-old retired schoolteacher who never married. For the past ten years, our mother, Shirley, ninety-two, has lived with Mary. When my sister wanted to take a fourteen-day Hawaiian vacation, she asked me to stay with Mom. How could I say no? She's been such a trooper. In two days, I realized how forgetful Mom had become. She put on a blouse and forgot her skirt. She used hand lotion instead of toothpaste. When Mary returned, I mentioned these oddities to her, and she merely replied, 'Bill, everything's fine. Don't worry.'"

"Two months later," Bill continued, "I received a call from Dale, Mom's doctor. Since he and I went to high school together, he always kept a special eye on Mom. 'Bill,' he told me, 'your mother needs more care. She's lost weight, her blood pressure is out of control, and she's developed a yeast infection on her chest, probably because she's not bathing. She appears confused and, most telling, she didn't recognize me. Bill, you need to talk to Mary. She denies anything is wrong.'"

"So," Bill said to me, "that's why I'm here. I'd like to see your facility before I bring Mary. I'll do a better job preparing her if I can describe what I've seen with my own eyes."

The following afternoon, both Bill and Mary arrived at my office. Looking tired and frightened, Mary loyally tried to cover for her mother, saying she had no problems with dressing, bathing, or memory. But as I questioned Mary, a different picture emerged.

"Tell me, Mary," I ventured, "how does your mom spend her day?" Mary did not respond. "Would she remember what she had for dinner last night?" I continued.

Mary laughed a little and said, "Well, no."

"Is she able to take her pills by herself in a timely manner?"

"No," said Mary, "I dispense all her medications."

"Could your mother tell me whether she took her pills today?"

"No," said Mary, growing visibly upset. "Mom's a little forgetful, but it's not like she has Alzheimer's or anything. She and I do just fine."

At this point Bill broke in and said, "Mary, you have to be truthful. Mom can't sit still for five minutes; she's right by your side asking the same questions over and over again. And because she needs too much for one person to provide, things aren't good between you and Mom anymore. I don't mean to make things difficult for you," said Bill sadly, almost in tears, "but I do know our mother needs more care. I'm sorry."

Because of Mary's inability to see reality, she perceived Bill's recommendation as criticism. As she listened, she became angry and defensive. "You don't think I've done a good job caring for Mom, do you Bill?" she said flatly. "Well, Mom and I are fine."

In denial, Mary believed that since she could deal with any problem her mother had, there was nothing wrong. In reality, she was placing her mother's health and her own in jeopardy. It took three months for Bill, with the help of his physician friend, to convince Mary that her mother needed more professional care.

The Spouse in Denial

"Your father drives just as he always has."
"Your mother and I are fine where we are."
"Anyone could get lost in this neighborhood."
"I can handle it."

After an adult child recognizes his parent's illness or dementia, the next denial to deal with is often that of the caregiving spouse. Fortunately, many adult children understand they are already losing one parent to illness or dementia, and will fight to keep the caregiving parent healthy and safe so as not to lose both.

I received a visit from Matt, a patent attorney, who was visibly upset about his parents. He and his brother and sister had been shocked into reality by their mother's heart attack, which had revealed a hidden side of their parents' lives.

"Whenever we inquired how she and Dad were doing," said Matt, "Mom would say, 'Don't worry about us.' At eighty-three, Mom had been in good health. But Dad is eighty-six and suffers from diabetes and dementia. The three of us, Lonnie, Hal and myself, live in the same state, each an hour from our parents. We're pretty good about visiting and felt we were keeping an eye on them. But last Sunday, everything changed. When I arrived at the emergency room, there was Dad, just sitting and crying in the waiting room. I didn't know whether to calm him down or check on Mom. In the next few hours, Hal and Lonnie arrived. Mom was admitted to the ICU for observation for two days. Since Hal had to work Monday morning, and Lonnie has three children in school, I volunteered to stay at home with Dad.

"The next two days were the longest of my life," Matt continued. "Without any idea of Dad's true condition, I found myself helping him shave, dress, and brush his teeth. Prescription bottles were scattered in the kitchen, bathroom, and bedroom. I had no idea when to give him his medicine. How could Mom have kept this from us? According to her, everything had been fine, and we didn't need to get involved. Even though it's obvious Mom and Dad can no longer live alone, we are totally unprepared for this."

Spouses Use Denial Differently

Spouses are the long-distance runners when it comes to caregiving. Many not only have strong feelings that this role should continue to the end, but they also have a tendency to cover up for the needy partner and deny the extent of the problem as a way of protecting the spouse. The caregiving spouse may walk a fine line with the rest of the family. On one hand, she doesn't want to push her children away; on the other, if she shares too much information, the kids may start telling her what to do. No parent wants to be told to give up the car, to hire help, or to move, but a husband or wife who can no longer give adequate care may place the spouse in jeopardy from what we call "benign neglect," a gentle phrase for doing all you're physically capable of even though it's not enough for the safety and welfare of the spouse.

In my experience, it is harder for the wife to accept help. With many years of caregiving already under her belt, she cannot admit that she is unable to give her husband the care he needs. Because she expected to take care of her partner for the rest of her life, she has made no contingency plans whatsoever. Many spouses have been in these relationships fifty, sixty, and even seventy years—a lifetime. To them the phrase "till death do us part" was a serious commitment. Many spouses have cried and said to me, "I can't abandon him. He wouldn't abandon me." Sadly, the burnout rate for caregivers is tremendously high, and many end up in the hospital along with the ailing spouse. According to Shirley Rose Tyson in her book *Geronto-logical Nursing Care,* "It is not uncommon for a caregiving spouse to die before the patient, due to the enormous physical and mental stress." Thus, a delicate battle ensues between the children's attempt to save the healthy parent and the caregiver's attempt to retain control over her life and marriage.

Coping with Denial

We each have a unique role in the family, and we each harbor differ-ent fears: the aging process, the loss of a parent's companionship, changes in family dynamics, loss of control, loss of independence, the embarrassing debilities of old age, terminal illness—the list is endless and personal. As we watch our mother or father slip away, fear percolates beneath the surface. Initially, denial slips in to help us cope with the fear and to allow us to regroup emotionally. However, at a certain point we need to wake up to the reality of our parent's condition and focus on both immediate and long-term needs.

Recognizing the subtle signs of decreased attention or mobility may be a new experience. Look at the checklist at the end of this chapter. Do any of these statements sound familiar?

CHECKLIST
Do you find yourself or family members saying the following things?

- My mother doesn't have Alzheimer's, but...
- Dad has a few problems—nothing out of the ordinary.
- Mom doesn't need outside help; we take care of our own.
- She's done one or two odd things, but nothing to worry about.

- There's no dementia in our family. He's just a little confused today.
- I see no reason to talk about this.
- It's just the normal forgetfulness that comes with age.
- I am just too overloaded right now, but your dad and I will be fine.
- You're being an alarmist.
- Mom has always been like that.
- My parents aren't really that bad.
- As long as I can handle his behavior, it's not a problem.

4 ⤳ PARENT-CHILD ROLE TRANSFER

When I was sixteen, my mother used to say to me, "When you're a parent, you can make the rules." At fifty-two, I was making the rules for her and I didn't like it as much as I thought I would. Our roles gradually reversed as I found myself taking the following actions:

- I asked my parents to call me when they got home from visiting to be sure they arrived safely.
- I accompanied them to doctor appointments.
- I replaced their toaster that hadn't worked for two months.
- I arranged for a cleaning lady to clean their home twice a week.
- I bought their food while I did my own grocery shopping.
- I became nervous when I hadn't heard from

them for two days and began to call daily to check on them.

- I bought a seven-day pillbox for my dad and began to prepare it weekly.
- I invested in an emergency-response system for them.

None of us expects to become the decision maker for our parents or to care for them as they grow frail. Having our parents depend on us is new. When the inevitable role reversal, or role transfer, takes place, it can be a complex and awkward adjustment. Although you may always feel like their little boy or girl, the burden of parent-like responsibility and decision making is gradually transferred to you—hopefully with their consent. Regardless of how sensitive and thoughtful you are, this process is not likely to go smoothly. Neither you nor your parents will be quite sure how to react. Just as they were unable to solve all our problems, so we will be unable to solve all theirs.

Ginger, Max, and Linda. Ginger and Max arrived in a taxi from the airport to meet their sister, Linda, at my office. Three weeks earlier, their father had died unexpectedly, leaving their eighty-eight-year-old mother alone. "We're not prepared to leave Mom on her own," Linda began. "She and Dad lived in the same house for twenty years, but it's too big for her now. Ginger and I feel it's time for Mom to sell the house. We think assisted living would be perfect for her."

As they spoke, I began to suspect that although her children were springing into action with the best of intentions, their mother had not been consulted. I asked them if this was so.

"That's why we came to talk with you," Ginger answered. "After we see a few facilities, we're going to talk with Mom."

"I feel your sense of urgency," I began, "but the rush-to-fix attitude, although well meant, may unintentionally make your mother feel she has no control over her life. As adult children, we may rush to make decisions for our parents so we can feel that everything is settled, but as long as your mom is competent, it is her decision to make. If you can help her maintain control over her current lifestyle, it will strengthen her independence and in the long run benefit each of you."

"But we're worried about Mom," said Max. "We don't want to be intrusive, but she just can't live alone. What about her finances? Should she still be driving? Isn't it our responsibility to step in? Ginger and I don't live in the area, so we want to leave Mom safe and settled."

"Max," I said, "your concerns are valid, but making all her decisions for her may not be the answer. Find out what is important to her. Does she want to remain in her own home? How much help will she accept? Does she want to keep driving? Talking about these issues will let your mother feel that when a change is necessary, it is her choice rather than yours."

Adult children feel overwhelmed and trapped by enormous life changes. So do their parents. Adult children feel sad and anxious about the future. So do their parents. Parents fear losing their independence. Adult children fear the burden of caregiving. If you can recognize that you and your parents are going through a similar process, the shared fear and uncertainty can build a stronger bond between you as you help one another answer questions together.

Role transfer is difficult for elderly parents for many reasons. Not only do they often experience loss of control over mental clarity and physical ability, but since they are used to seeing themselves as caregivers and decision makers, they also face a loss of identity. They may now have to rely on you to carry out their life decisions. Most disconcerting of all, they may have to make new living arrangements, after being in the same home for decades.

A Difficult Transition for an Adult Child Caregiver

There are many reasons for the emotional roller coaster caregivers go through.

1. **We are not prepared for this.** Michael lived in San Diego and drove to West Los Angeles every four weeks to visit his eighty-six-year-old mother, Betty, who lived alone. "When I visit Mom," he told me, "I take her out to an early lunch. I'm usually back on the freeway by three-thirty before the traffic hits." Michael had arranged for a companion named Maria to visit Betty twice a week, so he thought things would be under control while he took a two-month sabbatical in Italy. "When I returned," Michael continued, "the house was dark and the curtains were pulled. Mom looked awful and didn't know who I was. I called Maria and asked what was going on. Maria responded that following a doctor appointment three days earlier, Mom told her she no longer needed to take her medication for diabetes, so Maria removed them from the pill container."

Michael rushed his mother to an emergency room. "Stella, her blood sugar and her blood pressure were off the charts," he said. "But her confusion scared me the most. She wasn't even speaking in complete sentences. The doctor looked at me accusingly and said, 'Michael, you know your mother has suffered from pinpoint strokes for two years.'

"I didn't even know what pinpoint strokes were," said Michael.

"I asked the doctor why he never bothered to discuss it with me, and he answered, 'I spoke to your mother several times about this. She assured me you were informed.' Stella, Mom never told me. She's always swept bad news under the rug."

Within forty-eight hours, Betty's blood sugar and blood pressure were stabilized. Her confusion and disorientation were another story. "They're ready to send her home," Michael told me, "but how can Mom go home? She doesn't even know she's not home now."

Michael had never considered his mother living anywhere but in her own house. "How can I make decisions for her? She never told me she was in trouble. How was I supposed to know?" He clenched his jaw in an attempt to control his emotions. The pressure of seeing his mother in her frail, dependent condition and becoming her decision maker was overwhelming. Michael was not prepared.

2. **We feel trapped by new responsibility.** Millions of us who travel down this road have felt trapped. For many, the past two decades have been spent caring for dependent children. Now we find that caring for a dependent parent lies ahead, perhaps for another decade or more. This is not how we pictured our retirement.

My own role transfer began slowly. While every week added another small responsibility to my role as my parents' caregiver, our lives remained relatively the same. A phone call changed everything. "Stella, you'd better come over," my mother said. "Something is wrong with your dad."

Recently retired at the age of seventy-eight, my dad was a self-employed optician and worked six days a week. His work gave him a sense of purpose. I had quipped, "Dad will die the day he stops working." Four months after he retired, things changed, but not the way I expected. Dad remained physically strong; it was his brain that was dying.

When I arrived, my father was sitting on the couch, crying, a look of fear in his eyes. For the first time, he looked old to me. "I don't know why I'm crying," he said. "I'm scared. Your mother doesn't understand, but I'm scared."

At that moment, my role as a child was pulled out from under me. None of my years of professional experience had prepared me for this. My emotions during the next days ranged from sadness and anger to panic and fear of being trapped.

This isn't right, I thought, This shouldn't be happening to my dad. The sudden frailty of the man I had adored all my life was bewildering. I should have known better; I have seen clergy, psychiatrists, and even bereavement specialists immobilized when their parents' health failed. I had thought, How could this be? These people are the experts! But education and experience are no buffer for this life-changing moment. It is impossible to understand until it happens to you.

3. **We fear our parents' anger.** Harvey, ninety-three, had been a controlling father figure to Sandy all her life. "He demanded respect," Sandy said, "and he got it." As an only child, she was terrified of making decisions for her father. But Harvey, who managed his own estate, started to make financial mistakes. Then he had two car accidents and forgot to pay his medical insurance, which took weeks to resolve. When Sandy offered to help, her father made it clear he would not turn over any responsibility to her. Finally, Harvey began losing weight, stopped answering the phone, and believed people were after his money. Managing

his financial holdings remained important to him, although he was no longer able to do it responsibly. When Sandy came to see me, she was in turmoil, walking an uneasy line between offering assistance and taking charge. "If I do nothing, things will get worse. But if I bring up his finances, he gets angry. What do I do now?" she asked.

"You need emotional support, Sandy," I answered. "A place to vent your feelings. Have you considered joining a support group?"

"How would that help me deal with Dad?" she asked

"Support group members have been in situations similar to yours," I said. "By sharing your stress and confusion with the group, you will find that you are not alone. Many people are not comfortable sharing frustration and anger with family members and friends for fear of being judged. But in a support group, it's easier."

When I saw Sandy two months later, she had joined a support group.

"It was a good feeling to know others were going through a similar rough time," she told me. "I don't feel alone anymore. Not only have members shared what they've done right, but they were also brave enough to share what they've done wrong. We give each other advice and laugh about our frustrations. I don't feel as guilty anymore."

As Harvey's condition continued to fail, he required a twenty-four-hour caregiver and Sandy began making decisions for him. "He still gets mad at me," she said, "but I know I'm doing the right thing. The group has taught me not to personalize his anger. I've turned into a better caregiver."

"I" Statements. Simone, a Florida attorney, hired a geriatric-care manager to help her care for her ninety-year-old mother, Jane, who lived in Los Angeles. She's the reason I moved to Florida," laughed Simone. "Mom has a very strong personality, and I've never been good at dealing with her." Jane had been living at Sunset Village Assisted Living until she fractured her hip. Now temporarily in a nursing home, she did not like being told what to do and was becoming withdrawn and depressed. "I'll never get out of here," she told her physical therapist. To return to her beloved Sunset Village, Jane needed to be able to use a walker, but for two weeks she had been refusing to see the physical therapist, saying she was too tired.

"Do you think Mom will ever return to Sunset Village?" Simone asked me. "We can't pay for both places indefinitely. But if I tell her she's running out of money, she won't listen to me. She's very stubborn."

"Simone," I said, "when you address your mom using 'you' statements, it automatically sets her up to argue. Try using 'I' statements. Try saying, 'Mom, I'm worried about your finances. Keeping your room at Sunset Village and paying the nursing home is draining your savings. I'm concerned you won't be able to live where you choose if your money is gone. If you are not walking in three weeks, I need you to let me know that I should let the room go at Sunset Village.' It may cause her to respond to you as a daughter in need."

Phrased this way, it became Jane's decision, and Simone wasn't placed in a position of dictating terms to her mother. After three weeks and many hours of physical therapy, Jane was able to return to Sunset Village.

I have repeatedly seen "I" statements produce a win/win situation. Adult children are able to help their parents without disempowering them. Parents feel more control making their own decisions. Here are more examples of "I" statements:

- Mom, I'm worried that you haven't seen the doctor about your shortness of breath.

- Dad, if I'm not involved in your health-care plans, I'm afraid I'll be left alone to figure it out if you ever get sick.

- Dad, I feel unsettled that I'm not up to date on your finances. I wouldn't know how to manage if you had to go to the hospital.

- Mom, I'd feel a lot better if you'd let me do this for you.

- Dad, I need us to be partners in deciding about your safety and health; I don't want to guess what you'd want.

- Dad, I'm concerned something will happen to you if you drive.

4. **We may not be able to go to our parents for advice and approval.** A successful children's book author told me, "My latest book has been chosen for a prestigious award. The story is based on Mom's life, but when I showed her the book and expressed my excitement, she wasn't able to grasp the significance. She had always been my biggest cheerleader, encouraging me to be a writer, and I guess I just wanted her to be proud of me."

"In his days as a real estate attorney, my dad gave valuable advice to hundreds of people," Ben, a professor of anthropology, told me. "Whenever I needed information on buying or selling property, I always went to him. My wife and I are in the middle of selling an apartment complex, and it's getting complicated. It hurts that I'm not able to talk things over with him anymore."

When we were children, our parents guided our every decision. As we matured, their advice, welcome or not, provided a sense of security. Although they may not be the sound source of advice they used to be, remember, it still means the world to them to be asked their opinion; it gives them a sense of value. Even in a state of dementia, they will feel needed and appreciated. It is a kindness and courtesy not often extended.

5. **Our parents' aging mirrors our own.** "I've come to terms with my father dying," began Ken as he sat in my office. Two weeks earlier, his eighty-six-year-old father had had a stroke. "What's scares me is looking at Dad lying in the hospital bed; I can't stop thinking, That's me in thirty years."

When roles shift between you and your parents, you begin to identify with them and face your own mortality. Will you develop dementia as your mother did? Will your husband suffer multiple strokes as his father did? Will you lose your vision to macular degeneration? Will your husband need open-heart surgery? A glimpse of the future is one of the last lessons your parents teach you.

Fears of the Older Parent

"My husband and I need to feel in control. It's our bodies, our lives, our minds. Why does my daughter think it's time to take control of us?" —Amelia, age 78

To understand the fears and concerns our parents experience, I went to the source. As one elderly resident put it, "So you want the answer from the horse's mouth. Well, this filly ain't what she used to be." These are the six biggest fears residents have shared with me.

1. Fear, not of dying itself, but rather of the process of dying.
2. Fear of illness and pain.

3. Fear of being a burden, physically or financially.
4. Fear of being abandoned and alone.
5. Fear of "losing my mind."
6. Fear of losing independence.
7. Fear of being forgotten.

Claudette. At eighty-nine, Claudette is very engaging and outgoing. "My biggest fear," she said, "used to be dying before my husband; the children would never have known what to do with him. Now my big fear is major illness—I'm chicken. So far, other than having my children, I've only been in the hospital for gallbladder surgery. I told my family, I don't want to be hooked up—no tubes! If I'm really honest, my biggest fear isn't dying, because that will happen no matter what I do, but I don't want to linger, be a burden to my children, maybe even cost them money. That would be awful."

Charlie. Charlie, eighty-seven, is a salty, occasionally aloof individual, who has traveled and lived in many countries. Initially, Charlie said his biggest fear was outliving his money. But as we kept talking, he added, "My daughter is raising three children alone. All she needs is one more burden. That's why I moved to assisted living without much of a fight. She has a full plate, as it is." When I asked him if he was afraid of death, he answered, "Nope, but I am afraid of losing my mind." When we started to talk about dementia, Charlie ended the conversation.

Beryl. Beryl is a tall, elegant woman who used to be a fashion model; even at ninety-three, clothes and fashion are extremely important to her. She has a son, George, who hired a geriatric care manager named Sally to act as liaison between him and Beryl. Sally visits Beryl weekly to monitor her well-being and take care of any personal needs she may have. Beryl shared very private fears with me. "My son, George, lives in Europe and travels extensively. He loves me, probably a lot, but he's never here. I am really afraid of being alone and dying alone. I've had a very full life, I traveled, and I was married twice. Did you know I was also a pharmacist? I've had many friends but have outlived them all. When I die, no one will know who I was. That scares me. Being alone is no good."

Begin a Dialogue

Our parents have experienced many losses—the deaths of a spouse, siblings, and friends—and then their own physical decline. We can only imagine the fear and uncertainty they feel. As you assume new responsibilities and share decisions with your parents, there will be a few bumps in the road. Keep in mind the difficult emotional journey they are taking. As soon as possible, begin a dialogue with your parents and share your concerns. They may not want your help now, but as their health and abilities decline, they will need it. Talking it over ahead of time will take the pressure off the eventual transfer and make it a more comfortable process.

As our caregiving roles change, we will find our parents in need of guidance, decision making, physical assistance, possible financial support, and unconditional love—all of which we will offer. But as we perform parentlike tasks for them, and as life gradually strips them of everything they have, we should never take away the respect and honor due them as our parents. A guide we may become, but a substitute parent—no.

5 🍃 REDEFINING SIBLING ROLES

"It's me again...Bob Sherman," said a tentative voice on the phone. Bob had visited our nursing home twice, once to tour the facility, and again to gather more information. "Can you meet with my sister Jen and me tomorrow?" he asked. "We're ready to make arrangements to admit my mom."

Promptly at ten A.M., Bob arrived alone. He reminded me that Ann, his eighty-nine-year-old mother, had lived by herself for the past twenty-eight years. During the last two years, she had required more and more help from him. According to Bob, "Mom and I were doing fine. Then suddenly, my unpredictable sister Jen shows up and wants to take over Mom's care. But she hasn't been involved in Mom's life for years." Bob looked at his watch. "It's ten twenty-five—she's never on time." When Jen arrived minutes later, the tension between the siblings was palpable. It was difficult to find an issue they agreed on. Jen wasn't even sure that moving her mother was a good idea.

"She's going to move, Jen," Bob said tersely. "She needs more care than you know."

"Then I want Mom to see her room before she moves in," answered his sister. "She should help decide what furniture and pictures she wants. I'll bring her tomorrow."

The following morning, Jen and her mom arrived as planned. As the two of them looked around Ann's new room, Jen asked, "Mom, what about a television?"

"Your brother has one for me," said Ann.

"Mom, that's an old TV. I'll buy you a new one. The color and sound will be much better. You've chosen too many pictures, Mom; we need to narrow them down." Remembering a favorite picture her father had given Ann many years ago, she said, "There's one in Bob's living room, Mom. I'm going to tell him it really belongs here with you."

"I wish you two would get along," sighed Ann. "Everything is such a struggle. I feel like a referee." Looking at me in exasperation, she shook her head and said, "Siblings!"

Research consistently shows that in a majority of families, one member is designated primary caregiver and decision maker. As a family begins caring for an aging parent, traditional roles begin to shift. Rivalries hidden for many years resurface. Brothers and sisters who had good relationships find themselves at odds in matters of caregiving. I have seen families literally torn apart over the care of an aging parent.

Initially, some jostling for position in the family hierarchy may take place. Adult children may volunteer for caregiving duties and then later decline. But all family members must acknowledge what they can and cannot do. Ultimately, one steps up to the plate. Sometimes geography is the deciding factor. Occasionally the parent will decide.

If the youngest child becomes the primary caregiver, the "baby" is suddenly the leader in the family dynamic, telling older siblings what to do. This reversal can upset the traditional family order and cause considerable upheaval among the other siblings. The entire family should attempt to remain a team whose job is to agree on and carry out a plan that delivers quality care for the remainder of the parent's life.

Be Part of the Solution, Not the Problem

"Last evening, my sister Lisa stopped by as I was racing to my fourth grader's Back-to-School night," lamented Jennifer. As soon as Lisa saw the TV dinner I had given Mom, she started in on me. 'How can you feed Mom this junk?' she exclaimed. 'She should be eating organic food.' I was rushed, tired, and in no mood to defend myself. Once a week, Lisa visits to critique my caregiving, but she has never offered to shop, cook, or take Mom to the doctor."

Siblings not in the primary caregiving role deal with their own set of emotions. Some feel left out. Others are jealous about not being the "special" caregiver. Still others are sure their parent's care is not handled properly, yet are more comfortable instructing the caregiver on what to do while avoiding personal responsibility. Whether Lisa's remarks were a criticism of Jennifer or just a need to feel involved in her mother's care is not the issue. What matters is that her remarks did not contribute to her mother's care.

If you are not the primary caregiver, *do not wait to be asked for help*. For many reasons, caregivers are often reluctant to seek assistance. If you do not agree with the way your sibling is caring for your parent, decide whether you would want to step in and take over the caregiving responsibility. If you don't have the time or ability to provide the care yourself, you must accept your sibling's capabilities.

What You *Can* Do as a Secondary Caregiver

If you are a secondary caregiver not contributing physical care, find out what the caregiving costs are. Needless to say, monetary help is almost always needed and will certainly be appreciated. If you can't contribute money, offer a service such as laundry, housekeeping, or doing your parent's taxes. Acknowledge and show appreciation for the primary caregiver; positive communication between siblings can lighten difficult days. Always make sure the caregiver gets days off and vacations. That may mean you will have to be willing to sit in for her. Should the primary caregiver's health fail, it will throw the whole family into turmoil. (See Chapter 9, Burnout.) Thank-you cards and phone calls to show appreciation mean a lot to a busy caregiver. If your family has hired full-time or part-time caregivers, thank-you gifts will show you recognize their helpful efforts as well. Be creative. And if you are arriving from out of town to see your parent, remember that the situation is working, or you wouldn't feel free to "just visit."

Conflicting Directions to the Health-Care Staff

Marlin, an assertive movie producer, and Loretta, his equally assertive younger sister, were arguing as I walked into my office. "My brother and I are trying to make decisions about Mom's medical care once she joins you," Loretta began. She and Marlin had visited with me the previous week regarding their eighty-eight-year-old mother, Theora. Although Theora had been living on her own in a condominium for the last three years, both siblings agreed their mother now needed more help and supervision. However, their views differed on how this was to be accomplished. Even the date of admission was a point of dispute.

"Mother suffers from rheumatoid arthritis," said Marlin. "When she joins you, we'd like the staff to ask the doctor for a routine order of a pain medication."

"No," Loretta objected. "I don't want Mom 'drugged out.' Those medications aren't good for anyone."

"But I want to take Mom out on Sundays," said Marlin. "If she's in pain, she won't go. And family outings are good for her."

"Mom shouldn't even leave the facility for at least a month," Loretta stated. "She'll need time to acclimate to her new environment."

Although Marlin and Loretta both cared about their mother, each gave the nursing staff contradictory dos and don'ts for her care. Making the facility a battleground for unresolved issues between siblings can jeopardize a patient's health care. Whether there are two siblings or ten, choose *one* to act as a spokesperson for the family. Health-care professionals need to clearly understand family health-care decisions, and if they receive conflicting calls from family members, their cooperation may diminish.

It's Not About You. It's About Your Parent

"My sister Claire and I have had little to do with each other for years," Jaimie confided in me. "Before Dad died ten years ago, he provided for Mom financially, and I have pretty much watched over her since then. In the last few weeks, Mom has fallen three times, and it's just not safe for her to live at home anymore. Mom and Dad appointed Claire and me as coagents having power of attorney for health and finances. That requires us to act jointly. Even though Claire and I never agreed on much, we have to make arrangements for Mom's care."

"Before you make any final decisions," I cautioned Jaimie, "your sister should be with you. Let me give you a tour of the facility. Then come back and see me with Claire."

One week later, Claire arrived first. She was soft-spoken and comfortable exchanging information with me. On Jaimie's arrival, however, Claire stiffened. At first, each sister referred to the other in the third person. Claire was concerned about spending too much money for her mother's care, while Jaimie's philosophy was, "It's her money; spend it." Claire believed in conservative health care and that no heroics should be used. More proactive, Jaimie said she would consider certain medical procedures for her mother.

"You always want to be the decision maker," stammered Claire, "even though I'm the oldest."

"If you'd been around more," Jaimie shot back, "I wouldn't need to make all the decisions."

At that point I broke in. "The relationship you two share won't be resolved here today. The purpose of this meeting is your mother's care—she is the important one. Since you both took time to come to see me, I believe that at some level you are ready to work together."

Gradually, Jaimie and Claire began to understand that their relationship was secondary to their mother's well-being. As I worked with them on financial and health-care issues, some decisions were made easily, while others required flexibility and negotiation between the sisters. Months later, Jaimie admitted to me, "Mom and Dad knew my sister and I were different as night and day, but they also knew that we could cooperate to take care of them if we had to.

We still have our ups and downs, but working together as caregivers has made us closer."

The Primary Caregiver Can Feel Resentment

If you are a primary caregiver, prepare to feel resentment no matter how supportive your siblings are. It is normal to occasionally wish others were responsible instead of you. When you experience this resentment, try to let it go. Resentment becomes a major factor influencing what you do and how effective you are; it drains energy, immobilizes you, and takes up valuable time. You will need to conserve your mental energy and strength for the difficult tasks ahead.

The Lone-Wolf Sibling

"My brother isn't interested in helping."
"My sister never had a close relationship with our parents."
"My brother just said, 'Tell me when the funeral is.'"

"My brother sends money begrudgingly," said Roseanne, "but other than that, he's not there for our mother at all. I get so angry with him for not helping me when I know he could! I'm *not* the only child!"

"Roseanne," I asked, "would you do things differently if you were an only child?"

"Probably not. But I wouldn't feel so resentful," she answered.

"Then think of yourself as an only child," I urged her. "Thank your brother and go on with your life, because anger will only deplete your energy and productivity. Let your brother find his own comfort in the limited support he provides."

The hands-on caregiver makes adult decisions and difficult choices for her parent, experiencing parent-child role transfer on a daily basis. How other siblings experience role transfer depends on their involvement in the parent's care. For example, adult children who choose little or no involvement never have to deal with the reality of who their parent has become, or the real needs of an elderly parent with possible dementia. Those siblings have the luxury of remaining "children" until their parent dies.

A Plan for Role Transfer with Your Siblings

Effective caregiving requires a plan. Financial and health-care decisions will have to be made. Fortunately, a family meeting can provide a safe place to air feelings, to share concerns and opinions, and to take a good look at your parents' true condition. If you're lucky and your parents are still healthy, this is a good time to discuss and outline a plan of care. Even if your parents have already experienced a medical crisis that forces the issue, a meeting can prioritize your family's new health concerns. Here is a blueprint for a family conference:

- Limit the meeting to siblings and key family members who will be actively involved in your parent's care. Try to keep the number small. For those who cannot be present, set up a conference call or use a private chat room on the Internet. If anyone chooses not to participate, do not force the issue.

- Hold the initial meeting without your parent. That way you can discuss topics that might needlessly frighten or upset her. Address the most pressing health concerns your parent currently faces. If she is alert and able to participate in making appropriate decisions, invite your parent to the next meeting.

- Keep the meeting focused on your parent's care. You may need to involve a social worker, clergy, or geriatric-care manager as a facilitator.

- Arrive equipped to discuss topics of concern such as your parent's driving abilities and cognitive deficits. Allow each family member to speak without interruption or criticism.

- Be prepared to discuss your parent's legal, financial, and health-care needs.

- Designate a primary caregiver who will become the family decision maker. Discuss schedules and divide responsibilities to support the chosen caregiver. If financial support is needed, decide how this support will be divided among the siblings.

- Agree to read at least one book on the caregiving of aging parents so that everyone will have a more realistic idea of what caregiving entails.

- Avoid misunderstandings by remembering that each person can speak only for how he or she feels. I have noticed again and again that siblings are often unaware of one another's relationship with the parent.

- You won't settle everything in the initial meeting. Since the plan will continue to change as your parent ages, choose a date to meet again. At the next meeting, reevaluate to see if your plan remains effective for your parent's needs.

Hot Topics

Eventually, there may be uncomfortable subjects your family will have to discuss, such as the DNR (do not resuscitate) form, the appropriateness of hospice, the prolonging of life with feeding tubes, and the discontinuation of heroic measures. It is imperative that your parent designate a responsible person (often the primary caregiver) to have power of attorney for health care. If this legal instrument is not in place, and siblings are not in agreement, the health-care provider will follow the directions of the most "heroic" sibling. If five children choose "No heroics, do not resuscitate" and one chooses "Yes, resuscitate my parent," the care facility will follow the one who voices the most aggressive directive.

Siblings Who Are Enriched by Caregiving

The caregiving experience can be a source of family healing. The siblings who find a closer bond during this process are the ones who communicate and have a plan.

Before Morry placed his older sister Bridget with us, he could not abide the nervous, fluttering phone calls from his other sister Melanie. "Every time she called, I'd cringe," he said. Now, however, Morry and Melanie are working together as a team, caring for their older sister in her final illness. Dividing up the responsibilities, they decided Melanie would do more of the one-on-one "touchy-feely" relating to Bridget, which Melanie was good at, and Morry would make financial arrangements, empty the house, and close out Bridget's business. In separate meetings in my office, Melanie will say to me, "How is my brother doing?" Likewise, Morry will ask gently, "Is Melanie handling the pressure okay?" They came up with a plan to take care of Bridget that served both their needs and combined their strengths.

And for the first time in their lives, Melanie and Jack have a close relationship.

An Unequal Division of Care

One morning I received a call from Nancy, private secretary to a Mr. Thomas Thornton. Nancy explained that Mr. Thornton and his wife, Carmen, were attorneys who had worked together until last year when Carmen's health failed at age seventy-seven. After she fired four companions, Carmen's needs were more than her husband could handle; he opted for assisted living. "Mr. Thornton would like to place Carmen with you tomorrow," said Nancy. When I explained that it was necessary for me to meet with the family before I could admit Carmen, Nancy replied nervously, "He asked me to make all the arrangements for him. I'm not sure he has time to come in himself."

The following afternoon, Kristen, the youngest Thornton daughter, arrived to see me. "Dad's schedule is very tight," said Kristen. "I have four other brothers and sisters, but they're also busy professionals. I am the only one, as they put it, who 'doesn't work.' I have four children of my own and a hardworking husband, but I find time. During the past year as Mom's needs have intensified, I've tried to help her stay at home—but I can't do it alone, and everyone else has other responsibilities. I tried to convince my older brother to come with me today, but he just told me I knew what was best for Mom anyway.

"I know what's best for Mom," Kristen continued without a break, "because I'm the only one who does anything for her or tries to help her." Kristen began to cry, "I love my family, but I'm so angry. I don't like being totally responsible for Mom. I get so resentful. I just wish one of them would occasionally say, 'Let me help you.'"

If families unite, negotiate, and prepare for the inevitable needs of aging parents, the family structure stands a good chance of withstanding the stresses placed on it by this new stage in family life. Unfortunately, my experience has been that Kristen's situation, in which one family member assumes the entire caregiving role by default, is the most common.

A Plan Offers Control and Security

As our parents age into their eighties, nineties, and even one hundreds, sooner or later they will need assistance with day-to-day activities. Among siblings and other family members, good communication is vital for devising an effective plan of care. If a plan is ready to go into effect when needed, it will enable all family members to feel more in control and will eliminate many of the uncertainties of long-term care. It is never too early to start communicating.

6 ❧ UNFAIR PROMISES/ FAIR PROMISES

> *"I promised my mother I would care for Dad after she died."*
>
> *"Our family has always taken care of our own. I can't break my promise."*
>
> *"My father made me promise never to put him in a home, no matter what."*

We are all taught to keep our commitments, but what if keeping a promise means separating your parent from professional medical care? What if it means increased risk of a fall or mismanagement of medications? What if it means risking your own physical and mental health? These are all common results of hands-on, nonprofessional caregiving.

"Promise You'll Never Put Me in a Home"

"It's unfair," Lola said near tears, "for a daughter to have to choose a nursing home when her mother has instructed her never to do such a thing. But Mom's been to the hospital twice in the last month, first with aspiration pneumonia and dehydration; then she fell and hit her head on the corner of a table and had to go to the emergency room for sixteen staples to her forehead. Now, she's back at her house, but she calls me four or five times during the night. I'm getting tired and even resentful. I'm convinced she needs attention as much as physical care." Lola lowered her voice and confided, "I threatened her with a nursing home if she really needs me that often. I can't believe I did that to her."

However, the fact that she was now sitting on the other side of my desk showed that Lola was finally giving long-term care serious consideration. "It isn't just the promise to my mother," Lola continued. "My aunt Mabel is looking over my shoulder, too. She says the family has always taken care of our own. Stella, I just want to do the right thing. Between my own guilt and the pressure from family and friends, I feel paralyzed."

"Lola," I sympathized, "many of us promised never to place our parents in a nursing home. Frequently, this vow is made in better times when our parents can't imagine themselves in declining health and we can't comprehend the old-age disabilities they will face. Your promise may have been a loving one but—in the long run—it will cause grief and misunderstanding. If your mother had known years ago the anguish it would cause you today, I don't know that she would have asked for the promise."

"I'll take her home one more time," Lola said tentatively, then added, "but she can't continue this back-and-forth existence, in and out of emergency rooms."

Six weeks later, I received a phone call from a hospital discharge planner. Ethel had fallen yet again and fractured her right elbow and wrist. With her arm immobilized, she required assistance with bathing, dressing, eating, and going to the bathroom. Lola, telling her mother about our conversation, suggested she move into a nursing home just until her arm was functional again.

Two weeks after Ethel's admission, Lola stopped by my office. "Stella," she began, "I love my mom and I'd much rather be able to take care of her at home, but I'm so grateful for the care she gets here. Even though certain family members resent my decision, I'm finally sleeping at night. My family and my boss say I'm a nicer person to be around."

As caregivers, we face complex emotional issues that each family will approach differently. There is no right or wrong way. Taking care of an impaired elderly parent at home is a proper and loving endeavor. Consider, though, that a time may come when professional long-term care is the only safe solution.

Roberta and Helen

Roberta was the primary caregiver to her eighty-four-year-old mother, Helen. A successful psychologist, single parent, and mother of three, Roberta was going through a divorce and "just treading water" in keeping up with her demanding life. In my office, she explained that although her mother was mentally alert, she required assistance with bathing, dressing, and going to the bathroom. Two years earlier, Helen had been diagnosed with Parkinson's disease but chose not to accept the diagnosis even though it was confirmed by three physicians. As she required more and more care, she told Roberta, "Don't be thinking I need to be in some sort of home or anything! Remember you promised I could stay in my house."

"I don't know what to do," Roberta sighed. "Mom can't cut her own food anymore and even has difficulty bringing a spoon to her mouth. We were so grateful for Rosa, a full-time caregiver who was with Mom for nine months. But Rosa went to El Salvador for a visit and, five months later, she hasn't returned." A parade of caregivers followed. Two of the aides were not able to meet Helen's physical needs. A third seemed promising but left after three weeks. Still another had not been dependable, and the current caregiver had an unpleasant personality.

When an open sore from unattended cellulitis on Helen's leg became infected, she was admitted to the hospital with a high fever. Returning home five days later, Helen again ordered Roberta not to consider nursing home care. But the following week, Helen was back in the hospital, this time with a urinary tract infection. At this point, Roberta found herself in a dilemma. In view of Helen's medical and health needs, the discharge planner at the hospital recommended long-term care. Given twenty-four hours to find a facility, Roberta sat in my office crying.

"Now what do I do?" she asked. "Break my promise, or do what the hospital recommends?"

"Roberta," I said, "there is no guidebook to tell you when it's time to relinquish the care of your parent to others. But even a twenty-four-hour live-in caregiver cannot provide the care your mother needs. You made a promise you cannot keep."

"Yes, I've known it for some time now," Roberta replied. "Mom should have had more care all along."

"Roberta," I continued, "nursing home placement does not mean abandonment. It's a change, but you are still your mother's child, her chief advocate, companion, and support. A long time ago, you made a promise to your mother out of a sense of duty. In effect, you were promising to do the best you could. Now you must assure your mother you will still always be there for her."

Helen joined us the following day. Wanting to make her feel loved and important, Roberta brought her grandchildren to visit. At first Helen barely spoke to her daughter, but gradually she began to look forward to her daily visits. Two months later, Roberta e-mailed me: "Mom is coming around. Now she actually worries that I'm stopping by too often! The 'promise' is no longer hanging over my head."

Promises made years ago blind you to the realities of present needs and can immobilize you when you most need to make appropriate decisions. Having to choose a nursing home on twenty-four hour's notice can be nerve-racking; a good decision is nearly impossible. Think ahead. Prepare yourself for what may come. Even if you have to keep your research secret for now, investigate available options. Preplanning offers you control and better choices. It stabilizes a crisis during emotional times.

> **When asked to make a promise you're not sure you can keep, ask yourself WHAT IF . . .**
>
> *...your parent has a stroke or a fracture and can no longer walk unassisted?*
> *...your parent develops dementia and begins to wander?*
> *...your parent becomes incontinent of bowel and bladder?*
> *...you cannot find or keep quality caregivers?*
> *...your parent will not allow a caregiver in the house?*
> *...you fall ill and cannot give the support your parent needs?*

FAIR PROMISES

No one plans to place a parent in a nursing home. The parent doesn't want it, and neither do the adult children. But the fact is a majority of seniors will not live out their lives at home. What promises can you make to a parent who has flatly stated she will never leave home? Place yourself in her shoes. How would you like to be reassured and spoken to? Here are some fair promises you can safely make to your parent to reassure her of your commitment and love:

"I will never abandon you. If you ever need long-term care, I will be there to watch over you. To the best of my ability, I will ensure your comfort and care, and together, we will find solutions that work. I will always be an active voice for you."

"If you enter a nursing home, it will mean you are getting the kind of medical care I can no longer give you, but I will be there to oversee it. I will still be your child. You will still be my parent. And we will make the facility an extended part of our family."

"For the rest of your life, your happiness and safety will be a priority to me. With your welfare in mind, I will make the most responsible decisions I can for you. I will never place you in danger. Nor will I allow you to place yourself in danger."

Fair promises are harder to make than unfair promises, and they are even harder to discuss. It is easier to make an unfair promise: "Don't worry, I'll never put you in a nursing home." The conversation ends; everyone feels better. On the other hand, fair promises, although difficult to make, can reinforce your parent's sense of security and her need to remain included in the family. While she may not feel happy about it initially, fair promises will reassure her of your continued involvement in her life, and of your long-term commitment to her well-being.

7 🌿 "MY MOTHER DOESN'T HAVE ALZHEIMER'S, BUT . . ."

I have heard this statement thousands of times. In response, I gently inquire, "Can your mother describe what happened yesterday? Can she remember what she had for breakfast?" The answers are often no. As we start to discuss the cognitive abilities their mother has lost, a family member will quickly state, "Well, Stella, *my mother doesn't have Alzheimer's, but...* her memory is letting her down a bit."

While most people think of dementia as memory loss, it is the behavioral changes caused by dementia that bring people to my office. In fact, Alzheimer's has been described as a slow, progressive *disease of behaviors*. There is a wide variety of behavior exhibited by dementia patients, including becoming easily distracted or stuck in repetitive words and actions. In addition, you may notice restlessness, anxiety, depression, loss of inhibition, irritability, insomnia, apathy, delusions, hallucinations, and paranoia, as well as verbal and physical aggression. These behaviors may occur at any stage of dementia and often disappear as the disease progresses and new symptoms take over.

The word "dementia" has become an umbrella term for a variety of cognitive impairments. Alzheimer's is the most common form of dementia, followed by multiple infarct vascular dementia. Other major types being investigated are frontotemporal dementia, Lewy Body dementia, or dementia associated with Parkinson's.

Epidemic of the Twenty-first Century

Predicted to be the epidemic of the twenty-first century, Alzheimer's is a public health time bomb. Currently, Alzheimer's has immobilized 4.5 million Americans and has changed the lives of countless spouses, children, and friends. Today the average age at diagnosis is eighty and by age eighty-five, 45 percent of all seniors will display some form of dementia. Age, it seems, is the single greatest risk for Alzheimer's.

Although Alzheimer's disease has been recognized for more than thirty years, there remains a lack of understanding on the part of the clinical provider community. While geriatricians are trained in the diagnosis and care of patients with Alzheimer's, many primary care providers already in practice for many years have not received formal training.

Having personally experienced the heartbreak of two parents with Alzheimer's, I can sympathize with families I see who deal with this progressive, destructive disease. Both parents' diagnoses made me feel vulnerable, and I sometimes catch myself thinking, Will I get it myself? If I feel this way, how are other families coping? As diagnoses become more accurate, as medications become more effective, two things do not change: the inevitable cognitive and physical decline of the patient, and the emotionally wrenching and physically exhausting responsibility of the hands-on caregiver.

Patricia sank into the chair in my office, exhausted from the search for a facility for her husband, Tom. For six years, Patricia had been caring for Tom by herself. Now in the hospital, he was recovering from a fall, and his doctors had told Patricia he could not return home. Fearful and anxious, Patricia interrupted her story to say, "Stella, my husband doesn't have Alzheimer's—he just has dementia; you know, they're two totally different things."

What Patricia did not know was that regardless of her husband's diagnosis, it would not make a difference in the journey they were about to take.

Is It Really Alzheimer's?

Alzheimer's is a progressive, irreversible brain disease in which metabolism and chemistry in the nerve cells falter. In plain English, the brain cells die. Using state-of-the-art neurological and laboratory tests, a physician with dementia experience can almost always make an accurate diagnosis before death occurs.

Impaired memory is not always due to permanent downhill dementia. Other potentially reversible causes that your parent's doctor should look for include hypertension, thyroid disease, diabetes, urinary tract infection, alcoholism, and depression. A typical workup will include a urinalysis to rule out the possibility of infection and a blood test to rule out manageable or curable causes of disorientation. A CT (computed tomography or CAT) scan can rule out seizures or blood clots. An MRI (magnetic resonance imaging), which produces a more detailed analysis, can rule out strokes or brain tumors. A newer imaging test called SPECT (single-photon emission computed tomography) may increase the accuracy of an Alzheimer's diagnosis to nearly 100 percent by measuring blood flow to specific areas of the brain.

Psychological tests are frequently ordered to identify patterns that serve as clues to the nature of the underlying condition. For example, the Mini-Mental Status Exam measures the ability to handle simple tasks. It involves numbers, communication, recall of new and recent information, and the ability to process abstract thought. Your parent will be asked the year, the month, the season, and the name of the president. She will be asked to spell a word, and then spell it backward. The test takes a few minutes to complete, and it is easily scored.

Since clinical depression does not involve cognitive impairment, people with depression score higher on the Mini-Mental Status Exam than those with dementia. Often called pseudo-dementia, depression can mimic dementia by causing sleep disorders, weight gain or loss, memory impairment, confusion, and poor concentration.

My Father and the Mini-Mental Status Exam

When my father was well into stage two Alzheimer's, he had been hallucinating and twice had wandered away from home. His geriatric psychiatrist recommended that he be admitted to a geriatric-psychiatric unit. At the time, I was not dealing well with my father's dementia. I didn't care for the disease, I didn't care for his behaviors, and I didn't care for the doctor's recommendations. I was in serious denial. How could this happen to my dad? "If you want to see a crazy person," I said dramatically to the doctor, "just put my dad in a geri-psych unit, and you'll see a crazy person for sure." Only once in his life had my father been in a hospital and that had been fifty years earlier. The fearful look on his face as the doctor questioned him during the office visit worried me. I dreaded what his reaction might be when we admitted him to the hospital and left him overnight. Although I knew his behavior was out of control, the thought of Dad scared and alone was almost more than I could bear. With the help and reassurance of my brother Anthony, and with the doctor's guidance, we admitted my father to a geriatric-psychiatric unit that afternoon.

The admitting physician administered the Mini-Mental Status Exam. "Raul," he asked, "can you name the current president?"

"I know I don't like him," answered my dad.

"Can you count backward from ten to zero?"

"In Spanish or English?" he answered with a glint in his eye. My father was bilingual.

"Raul, did you graduate from high school?"

"Yes."

"What was the name of the high school?" I could see my dad trying desperately to come up with the correct answer. I wanted to help him. *Bowie High, Dad,* I kept thinking to myself, wishing he could hear me.

"The name," said Dad, "was the School of Hard Knocks." The only question my father actually answered correctly was that he had graduated from high school. Yet, well into second stage Alzheimer's, he was able to come up with meaningful, clever, and amusing answers.

All night I worried about him. At eight-thirty the next morning, Dad was not a happy camper. "Stella, I don't need to be here. Take me home!" he demanded, using his I-Am-Your-Father, Do-As-I-Say voice.

Resisting, I asked, "How did you sleep, Dad?"

"How can anyone sleep here?" he stormed. "The Chinese people were chopping, cooking, and partying all night. I think your mother was with them. I don't know why she does those things."

Then I realized Dad was where he needed to be. He remained in the unit seven days. During the last two days, the correct psychotropic drugs had taken effect, and he was no longer angry or anxious. To my amazement and delight, on the fifth day, I found him socializing with the other patients. Taking me by the hand, he proudly introduced the other residents on the floor as his optical patients who had come to consult him. In his mind, he was busy at work; he had mentally slipped into the safe world of his former profession.

His demons in check, my dad was able to return home. The quality of his life improved, as did ours. The geri-psych unit was the right choice for my father at that time.

"Your mother is eighty-five. What do you expect?"

Beware the physician who asks this question. Families interpret this to mean there is nothing they can do. Thus, the parent goes undiagnosed and does not receive proper care. Yet it is crucial to establish an early diagnosis for dementia. While Alzheimer's is not presently curable, there are medications that help control symptoms, improve functioning, and provide a longer time during which your parent can remain independent. This extra time gives the family the opportunity to plan the future and arrange a support system.

Early Diagnosis Is Frequently Delayed

Research suggests that the average delay in diagnosis of Alzheimer's is two years. Rarely does the patient seek medical attention for his own symptoms. Typically, when problem behaviors can no longer be denied, the family initiates the visit to the doctor. The usual reason is memory loss. Your parent's internist may recommend a geriatric psychiatrist or a neurologist. If you have an option, a geriatric psychiatrist would be my choice, because they deal more with behavior, and dementia is a disease of behaviors.

Looking for a Pattern

When do you take notice? What behaviors merit further evaluation? It is surprisingly easy to conceal problems related to dementia. The disease reveals itself in patterns, that is, in repeated behaviors not historically part of the personality. If your mother has misplaced her glasses since she was forty-five, this is not a behavior to worry about. However, a new behavior unusual for her may warrant concern.

Following are some of the common early patterns of Alzheimer's and other dementia disorders (which we called "red flags" in Chapter 2):

- Short-term memory loss; difficulty retaining new information
- Lost or misplaced objects
- Neglected household chores
- Poor personal hygiene
- Careless appearance
- Faulty judgment; unsafe decisions
- Noticeable repetition in conversation
- Minor car accidents
- Slight reduction in language skills
- Stale food or no food in the refrigerator
- Reduced interest in former hobbies, such as reading, knitting, or social outings
- Decreased interest in friends or family

While symptoms are developing, your parent will probably remain alert and social. Don't be surprised if he adamantly denies the above symptoms. But if he displays patterns that strike you as out of the ordinary, it is time for a physical and cognitive assessment to rule out inappropriate medications, depression, thyroid imbalance, or other conditions that mimic dementia.

Becoming Your Parent's Advocate

As time passes, your parent will require you to be an integral part of the health-care team; your input at the doctor's office will become critical. Keep in mind that your parents' generation was taught to ignore minor ailments. Asked how they are feeling, they have the bad habit of replying, "I'm fine, Doctor." So the more clearly you are able to articulate your parent's symptoms and behaviors, the more help you will be to the doctor. Since zeroing in on dementia is difficult at best in early stages, details are valuable. Try to pinpoint when you first noticed changes.

Behavior problems are awkward to discuss with the physician while your parent is present, since those behaviors you worry about may be exactly the behaviors your parent will deny. If possible, call the physician before the appointment to go over the reasons for the visit, or make an appointment and see him first without your parent. A conscientious doctor will appreciate the observations you can offer.

Some health-care professionals have divided dementia into as many as ten stages. Personally, I find the three-stage division to be more practical and understandable for caregivers. While each stage has symptoms and difficulties that overlap to some degree, I have consistently noted the following:

> *Stage One is hardest for the patient himself.*
> *Stage Two is hardest for the caregiver.*
> *Stage Three is hardest for the primary decision maker.*

There is no "typical" case of dementia; everyone experiences it in his own way. One may wander, another may not; symptoms from Stage One can appear during Stage Two, and vice versa. The following are short lists of common behaviors marking the three stages of Alzheimer's and related dementias. While it may be heartbreaking to read these lists, it is important for the family and caregiver to know what to expect in the years to come and to be prepared with a plan for all the "what ifs."

Stage One: Duration two to four years from onset of symptoms.

The hallmark of early dementia is persistent short-term memory loss.

He may be able to mask lapses in memory.

Your parent is usually still social and alert, although he may know "something" isn't right.

He will have poor concentration and difficulty retaining new information.

He may forget appointments and names.

He may put things away in the wrong places or leave the stove on.

He may forget to pay a bill or pay it twice; he is susceptible to money scams.

He may begin to withdraw from favorite activities.

He may get lost while driving.

He will begin to repeat stories or questions.

He may have problems naming common objects.

He may display moodiness or slight hostility.

Personal hygiene may slip a notch.

He may refuse to allow help in the house.

He may have difficulty calculating numbers, or finding specific words.

He may decide he does not need medication.

He may be anxious for no apparent reason.

He may be easily upset or depressed, often in response to the changes taking place.

He may exhibit anger at being confronted with any of the above.

Stage Two: Duration two to ten years—the longest stage.

Your parent will experience increasing memory loss and shorter attention span.

He will experience increasingly impaired judgment.

He will repeat stories and questions in a short span of time.

Minor dents to his automobile may progress to more serious accidents.

His appearance may be markedly unkempt.

He may get lost in familiar places.

He will have difficulty following more than one direction at a time.

His coordination, increasingly poor, will create a risk for falls and accidents.

His appetite may diminish.

He will require assistance with bathing, dressing, and possibly eating.

He may have increasing fear or suspicion of others; he may accuse a spouse of infidelity.

He may start to wander or pace.

He may lose items and claim they are stolen.

He may see or hear things that are not there.

He may become uncooperative, hostile, or aggressive.

His sleep may become disturbed; he may nap at odd hours and wander at night.

He may repeat meaningless tasks with greater frequency.

He may not recognize friends and family he doesn't see regularly.

He may begin to experience urinary incontinence.

He may spend more time in bed.

He may become restless in late afternoon or evening.

As dementia progresses, long-term memory will begin to fail.

Stage Three: Duration one to three years. Total Dependence.

> *He will eventually experience complete disorientation as to time and place.*
>
> *He may not recognize relatives and friends (or possibly himself in the mirror).*
>
> *He will need total twenty-four-hour physical care.*
>
> *He may lose weight even with a good appetite.*
>
> *He may have difficulty swallowing or be unable to swallow.*
>
> *He will need to be fed or he may stop eating.*
>
> *He will become totally incontinent.*
>
> *He will not be able to get out of a bed or chair unassisted.*
>
> *He will become noncommunicative, speaking in unrelated sentences or not speaking at all.*
>
> *At the end of Stage Three, he will be bedridden and asleep much of the time.*
>
> *He will become susceptible to malnutrition, infection, and pneumonia.*

By this point, difficult end-of-life decisions should have been made by either a spouse, an agent having durable power of attorney (see Chapter 24), or the mutual agreement of the patient's children. For example:

- Will a DNR (do not resuscitate) form be signed?
- Will antibiotics be used for all infections or only those that cause discomfort?
- When your parent has difficulty swallowing, will a feeding tube be used for nutrition? An IV for hydration?
- When is readmitting your parent to the hospital no longer in his best interest? (See Chapter 22, Time to Think About the Final Journey.)
- Is hospice appropriate?

Ultimately fatal, Alzheimer's and related dementias may last anywhere from five to seventeen years. Considering the wide range of symptoms, it is no wonder caregivers find themselves overwhelmed. A standard plan of care will not do for this disease; you must remain flexible and shift with your parent's changing needs.

How Much Should You Tell Your Parent? Camille, age one hundred, was well into stage two dementia. She still had good social skills, but often could not recall what happened five minutes ago as her memory came and went. Her eighty-year-old daughter, Sandy, had just suffered a stroke and did not want her mother told about it. However, Camille's nephew, a psychiatrist, felt it was the right thing to tell her the truth about her daughter. On hearing the news, Camille cried all afternoon and night, not eating dinner or breakfast. By the next morning, she was too weak to get out of bed. Strangely, by noon, Camille had forgotten about Sandy's stroke. But later in the afternoon, she remembered again, and for the rest of the day, cried so hard her doctor ordered an antianxiety medication. Every time she remembered, Camille grieved as though hearing the information for the first time.

Should You Tell Your Parent She Has Alzheimer's? Current medical literature supports the belief that every person has the right to be made aware of the diagnosis. If your parent is in early stage one Alzheimer's, she should definitely be told. Assured she is not "going crazy," she can participate in future choices by reviewing her will, her power of attorney, and her advance directives. Additionally, she can be made aware that there are medications available and research programs she might participate in. By sharing with her family how she wishes to be cared for and her preferences concerning end-of-life issues, she will have more control over her current and future life. Further, you can explain why driving or cooking would be dangerous. For the rest of the family, the open discussion allows a better understanding of the changes that are taking place and may deflect denial, blame, or misplaced anger.

However, suppose your parent is at a point where short-term memory comes and goes. I believe that to burden your parent with the news that she has Alzheimer's when she has lost the ability to process the information serves no purpose. In fact, telling your parent sad news of any kind at this stage may leave her in a painful limbo. So before you share this kind of information with your parent, think: Will she benefit from knowing? Or are you just telling her because you think it is the correct thing to do? Sometimes we have a responsibility to tell our parents; sometimes we have a responsibility not to tell.

"If I don't take action soon, I'm afraid I'll hurt Mom," sobbed Janice. For seven years, she had cared for her ninety-one-year-old mother at home. "Sometimes she's just plain mean," Janice continued. "When she needs her diaper changed, she screams and tries to hit me. If anyone else had to take care of her, they'd hit her back. To make matters worse, my husband is in a wheelchair from an accident at work, and now I have to do everything for him, too. He never liked the way Mom treated me, but now he wants her out of the house, and I can't blame him. He constantly reminds me I take care of her for free while I'm taking her abuse. Last night was the worst. I really lost it and began yelling at Mom. If the good Lord hadn't been with me, I would have hit her back and I don't know if I could have stopped."

I could feel the emotional struggle within her. "Janice," I warned her, "you are expending tremendous physical and mental energy without rest or appreciation. You are a textbook example of caregiver burnout."

Although caregiver burnout has undoubtedly been around for millennia, it was not defined in medical literature until recently. Perhaps not surprisingly, primary caregivers are as susceptible to depression and illness as the parents or spouses for whom they care.

The ages of caregivers range widely from thirty to ninety; they can be single, married, divorced, or widowed. While I have seen dependable granddaughters and reliable friends become caregivers, more commonly it is spouses, daughters, or daughters-in-law, in that order. With life expectancies inching higher every year, caregiving spouses are often in their eighties and nineties. When one parent dies, women traditionally provide much of the informal care for the remaining parent. Stunning statistics show that after the average American caregiver spends seventeen years raising a dependent child, she can expect to spend another eighteen caring for her dependent parent. Since women today often delay childbearing, there is an increased likelihood of an overlap between child rearing and caring for a parent.

Personality-wise, caregivers tend to be rescuing types. Often, they are sensitive, idealistic people attempting to manage all circumstances that involve their parents. Setting up unrealistic expectations for themselves, adult children may become so focused on meeting parents' escalating needs that they lose sight of the fact that there is no way to control the aging process. The result is unrecognized stress. They may hesitate to ask for help, fearing refusal will result in an unpleasant family confrontation. If you find yourself experiencing the following symptoms for more than two weeks, be aware they may affect your caregiving abilities and you may be headed toward caregiver burnout.

Physical Signs

Frequent headaches

Back or neck pain

Muscle spasms

Poor personal hygiene

Chronic fatigue or lack of energy

Disrupted sleeping patterns, including nightmares

Heart palpitations

Digestive problems, such as diarrhea, constipation, or nausea

Susceptibility to illness

Decreased interest in sex

One third of all caregivers describe their own health as fair to poor. In other words, they give care at the expense of their own well-being. If you are a caregiver, have you experienced chronic low-grade aches and pains? Are you constantly trying new drugs or alternative medicines to get more energy? Listen to your body. It is important that you begin to address your own needs before you suffer a breakdown or a serious illness.

Emotional Signs

Impatience

Anger, irritability, or resentment

Sadness or unexplained crying episodes

Inability to experience joy or happiness

Anxiety or guilt

Apathy or isolation

Mood swings

Forgetfulness

Loss of a sense of control

Feelings of hopelessness or of being trapped
Inability to concentrate or make decisions
Suicidal thoughts or the urge to hurt others
Inability to face another day
Feelings of failure

Behavioral Signs

Overreacting to criticism
Increased use of nicotine, alcohol, or drugs
Decreased productivity at work
Loss of interest in hobbies
No time for friends
Overeating or not eating enough
Refusing to take vacations

All these symptoms of burnout are also classic signs of depression.

The Hidden Patient

Denise arrived at my office weary and ready to break. "My father-in-law still lives in his own home," she explained, "but he's ninety and getting weaker and more forgetful. My husband, Joe, is convinced that if he goes over to his dad's house before and after work every day to do some chores and make sure he's eating, everything will be okay. Well, last night when he got home from Pop's, Joe was nauseated; then he got cold and clammy, like he was ready to faint. I drove him to the ER, where we sat for eight miserable hours before they admitted him with what they think is a bleeding ulcer.

"I haven't slept for twenty-four hours," she went on. "When I finally left the hospital at eight this morning, I stopped to check on

Pop before I went home. I found him on the bathroom floor and I could hardly get him up. Now what am I supposed to do?" Denise began to cry. "If Joe couldn't handle this, how can I? All three of us are going to end up in the hospital."

The effects of the caregiver's burden have been widely documented. By attempting to shoulder not only his own responsibilities, but also several of his father's, Joe became the "hidden patient." Since his expectations for the outcome of his dad's continued care were unrealistic, Joe was experiencing unrelieved stress, and he was unaware of the strain his body was undergoing.

Still crying, Denise added, "Joe and I had been planning to travel after we retire. I know it sounds selfish, but now we're chained to the routine of taking care of Pop."

"Denise," I said, "your concerns for yourself and Joe are real. Caregivers often fail to take care of themselves. Joe has to learn he can't do it all. He has to ask for help."

The good news is that burnout can be minimized and controlled. When I was caring for my own parents and feeling that I wasn't doing enough, I would stop and ask myself, "How realistic are my expectations?" This question helped me focus and set limits on what I could do. For example, my mother was invited for dinner every Wednesday. But when those dinners conflicted with a school function for my son or a business engagement with my husband, I would remind myself how much I did for my mother, not how much I *didn't* do. I knew Mom was in her apartment with Maria, her live-in companion, safe and cared for because of my planning. I tried not to invent guilt where it didn't belong. Here are some strategies that I hope will help you be a realistic caregiver:

- Get enough sleep.
- Visit your doctor for a checkup if you are not feeling well.

- Exercise to relieve tension, even if it's only walking around the block.
- Ask for help with specific tasks—shopping, parent sitting, etc.
- Learn to say yes if others offer help. If they do not do things to your satisfaction, let go of your controlling tendencies.
- Stay in touch with friends.
- Find someone you trust—a friend, professional therapist, or member of the clergy—with whom to discuss your feelings.
- Give yourself permission to be angry, but accept your limitations and deal with what is practical.
- Remember, it is okay not to know all the answers. There is no single, correct way to provide care.
- Arrange to take regular mini-breaks from caregiving.
- Make a detailed list of what you do for your parent and read it over when you think you are not doing enough. Give yourself credit.

Work Interruptions

Has caregiving significantly interfered with your job? Has it caused you to miss work? Caregivers who are also employed outside the home report more family conflict and more job stress than noncaregivers. Findings also demonstrate that caregivers who are employed use the phone excessively, make more mistakes, and have higher rates of accidents, tardiness, and absenteeism than noncaregivers.

Beverly had just been offered a promotion to senior vice president at her financial services firm. Sitting in my office, she explained her conflict. "The very same day, my mother's neighbor, Judy, called me from Chicago. I hadn't seen Mom for three months, but Judy always kept me up-to-date on her needs. Now she was concerned and felt I should fly out to check on her. When I arrived in Chicago, I discovered that Mom did indeed require more supervision. She needs to live near me now, which means moving her to Los Angeles. This is going to take a lot of organization, because I'm married and have two teenagers. I turned down the promotion; I just couldn't learn the new job while getting Mom settled with the care she's going to need. Career-wise, it was tough, but it has to be this way for my sanity."

"Beverly," I responded, "it may have been a difficult decision, but it shows sound judgment. You understood your limitations and put your own mental and physical health first. If you are not stable and focused, you will not be able to successfully relocate your mother or care for your family."

Adult children who care for older parents face sacrifices like Beverly's every day. Learn to say no and set realistic boundaries. If you keep your eye on what you *can* do, it will prevent you from being overwhelmed.

Waiting to Live

"I feel like I'm being held hostage by my mother's illness."
"My doctor doesn't understand."
"My friends don't understand."
"My husband doesn't understand."
"My brothers and sisters don't understand."

It is difficult for others to comprehend how exhausting and anxiety-provoking caregiving can be. As bystanders, they cannot fathom how the immediacy of caregiving overwhelms the rest of your daily life.

When was the last time you had fun? Has caregiving caused you to miss out on friendships? Are your children resentful of time you spend with your parent? And what about your spouse? Does caring for your parent leave you so tired you have lost interest in sex? It's difficult to be a fantasy in the bedroom when you're emotionally and physically drained by the demands of child care, parent care, and the workplace. Since caring for your parents can take you away from regular activities and responsibilities, balancing your time is crucial.

In order to take care of yourself, it is essential to get the support you need from family, friends, and professionals. This support is a requirement, not a luxury, and can range from financial help, assistance with meals, and adult day care to a paid companion or assisted living. Good relationships become strengthened when support systems are put in place. But you must speak up—people cannot be expected to guess your needs.

Social Isolation and Depression

Paul's mother, Rita, was eighty-two years old and had lived with Paul for ten years. They had shared a good, close relationship. All his life, Paul had looked forward to retiring and seeing the world, but about the time he was ready to retire, Rita started exhibiting peculiar behavior. She could not remember recent events. She became angry for no apparent reason. She began acting out inappropriately. By the time I met Paul, he was tired and resentful. "Right now my neighbor is sitting with my mom," he said, "but I can only be gone forty-five minutes, because it's not fair to ask him to deal with her longer than that. Nowadays, I rarely get to leave the house—we can't even go to church anymore. My brother says I have to do something."

Families, spouses, and friends may gently try to warn a caregiver that he is in trouble, but it is hard to see the forest for the trees. A caregiver totally enmeshed in the care of a parent loses sight of life outside the home. For caregivers of Alzheimer's patients especially, social isolation is common. When patients don't behave as appropriately as they used to, friends and family find it awkward to interact with them and may stop visiting. Perhaps as a result, caregivers are two to three times more likely to report symptoms of depression than noncaregivers and will use on average 70 percent more prescription drugs. Depression will not go away by itself while you continue to give care. If you harbor unrealistic expectations about yourself as a caregiver, you are at high risk for loneliness and isolation.

Depression can be a vicious cycle: You feel that it's useless to ask for help, and besides, you don't have time to go to the doctor. So you take no action. If you're a primary caregiver and you can relate to any of the symptoms listed in this chapter, you may be experiencing depression that would best be addressed by a health professional. Do yourself and your parent a favor—take the following steps:

- Make time to talk with your doctor and explain the situation.
- Join a support group of caregivers; even an online chat room can help.
- Consider a geriatric-care manager who will assess your parent's current needs and coordinate her care. Contact the National Association of Professional Geriatric Care Managers.
- Contact your local chapter of AARP or Agency of Aging;

they will tell you about services in your area, such as adult day care, caregiver support groups, and respite care.

• Contact health-related organizations such as the Alzheimer's Association or the Parkinson's Association for help in preparing yourself for the progression of the disease.

Take care of your own mental, emotional, and physical health. Your caregiving abilities depend on it. When you acknowledge your limits and accept help, it lifts the burden for everybody.

Alzheimer's and Burnout

Alzheimer's has been described as a disease of two people—the patient confined by the caregiver for his own safety, and the caregiver virtually imprisoned because the patient cannot be left alone. As Alzheimer's progresses over time, it taxes every level of physical and emotional life for the caregiver.

Spouses, who compose approximately 50 percent of all primary caregivers in dementia care, are the most susceptible to illness. Because stress and depression can permanently alter the responsiveness of the immune system, these spouses are at higher risk for heart attacks, high blood pressure, depression, and other diseases.

Nina, Ralph, and Burt. "How can I just leave him here and go home alone?" eighty-eight-year-old Nina lamented. "I've been married to Louis for sixty-eight years!" When a geriatric psychiatrist recommended that Nina begin looking for long-term care for her ninety-two-year-old husband, her sons Ralph and Burt brought her to see me.

"In effect, Dad has already been taken from us," said Ralph. "Now we need to protect Mom."

When the Alzheimer's developed to a difficult stage, Nina had managed with the help of a twenty-four-hour live-in aide. Now, Louis needed help walking, required feeding, and was incontinent of bowel and bladder. Most difficult of all, he was sometimes verbally abusive.

"The boys love us both and mean well, I know that," she said. "But how can I move Louis out of our home? I'd be abandoning him at the time he needs me the most. No one knows Louis like I do. He has to have warm milk before bed. He doesn't like the dark. And if I don't check him frequently during the night, he'll be soiled."

Burt added, "Mom has been waking up the aide every two to three hours at night to check on Dad. No one is getting enough sleep, and the aide is complaining to Ralph and me."

"Don't be concerned about my getting enough sleep," Nina said. "I just worry about Louis."

I asked Nina about her relationship with her husband, and she spoke about the former days, idealizing the relationship. "Oh, Louis and I have had no problems. After a lifetime of living together, we can anticipate each other's needs. Everything is fine." Then she paused, broke down in tears, and confided, "Everything is not fine anymore. Sometimes Louis says very cruel things to me. He doesn't mean them, but I get so sad and angry. And sometimes I get scared."

"What frightens you?" I queried.

"I just get so tired even with live-in help. I'm afraid I'll break down. Then who will take care of Louis?" Turning to her children, Nina said, "Boys, I haven't talked about this before, but lately my nights have been unbearable. When I sleep, I have nightmares. When I can't sleep, my heart pounds so hard it scares me. I haven't wanted to burden you with this."

"You can't handle this much stress alone," Ralph asserted.

"Mom, we'll do whatever it takes to help," Burt added as he stood up and hugged her. "We aren't ready to lose you, too."

"I'll be fine, son," she responded, placing her head on his shoulder.

Handing Nina a tissue, I explained to her that handing over the care of Louis would be one of life's most difficult transitions. As the World War II generation has aged, they have proven to be faithful and enduring caregivers. But, typically, these spouses in their eighties and nineties have had a difficult time recognizing when their own health was in jeopardy. In a recently published study of fifty-four thousand female nurses, it was found that a woman's risk of heart attack and heart-related death nearly doubled if she took care of her ill or disabled husband for at least nine hours a week.

"Mom," Ralph said, "we know you're dedicated to Dad, but you can't go on like this anymore. If something happened to you, Dad would have to go to a nursing home anyway, and then there wouldn't be anyone to visit him every day."

Shortly after our meeting, Nina was indeed found to be at high risk for heart attack. She was briefly hospitalized and received a pacemaker. With the emotional support of her children, she realized she could no longer provide the best care for Louis, and she placed him with us the following week. Despite a family's best efforts at home care, most Alzheimer's patients are eventually placed in nursing homes when their needs become too great or when stress threatens to overwhelm the caregiver.

Ask for Help *Now*

Caregiving can be a thankless and physically grueling job. While the stress of caring for a young child is offset by the anticipation of a bright future, caring for an aging patient holds no such hope. Caregiver burnout must be treated with compassion and awareness. Until you walk down that road, you will not understand the guilt, frustration, and exhaustion of trying to deliver adequate twenty-four-hour care to someone you love. Oddly, caregivers traditionally do not give themselves credit, because they never think they've done enough. If you are a primary caregiver, you must learn to care for yourself and start asking for help now.

10 🍃 THREE WAYS TO ENTER LONG-TERM CARE

There are three ways to enter long-term care: **medical crisis,** perhaps a stroke or serious fall; **invisible crisis,** a gradual decline in the ability to live independently; and **advanced planning,** in which families organize a transition to long-term care. It is my hope that by the end of this chapter, you will place yourself squarely in the "planning" camp and help change the crisis-driven mind-set that presently accompanies long-term care.

I. Medical Crisis

In my experience, roughly 95 percent of families inquiring about long-term care are in a state of crisis. Anxious and fearful, they venture into the unfamiliar territory of hospitals, rehab facilities, and nursing homes with no idea of what to expect. The unanticipated financial burden only raises the overall level of stress.

Joan, Katharine, and Ed. When Joan appeared in my office in Los Angeles, she was frantic about her parents, Katharine and Ed, who lived in New York. From three thousand miles away, she had been monitoring their lives with daily phone calls. Even though her mother was having cognitive difficulty, Joan had felt comfortable because her father was physically and mentally able.

But one day she could not reach them. After waiting twenty-four hours, she finally called their neighbor, who, unable to contact the couple, in turn called 911. When paramedics arrived, they found Ed on the floor, unconscious, the victim of a stroke. Nearby, Katharine sat silently watching him. Joan flew to New York. Now that her father was physically handicapped and unable to care for her mother, Joan realized there was no emergency plan.

She decided to relocate her parents to the West Coast, but the logistics of moving them, one physically handicapped, and the other mentally challenged, were mind-boggling. "Naturally," said Joan, "the plane was late, so they arrived at the nursing home at two in the morning. It was difficult for the staff to deal with their anxiety at being in this new, strange place."

The first three days were stressful for everyone. Except for her interview with me, Joan had never been to a nursing home, and was exhausted by the relocation process. Her parents had never been to a nursing home either. For the first time, Ed found himself in the role of a patient. He was alert, but nonambulatory and unable to speak. His wife, Katharine, couldn't understand what was wrong with him. Why wasn't he up? Why didn't he get lunch for her?

Although Katharine and Ed eventually adjusted to their new life, a medical crisis without a backup plan is not the recommended way to enter long-term care. Before a physical or a cognitive disability develops in your parent, run various scenarios through your mind.

Discuss the "what ifs" with parents and siblings and come up with a first draft of a plan. Whether you use it in two years or ten years, you will avoid a possible crisis or family disharmony. If you are likely to be the main caregiver, maintain clear lines of communication with other family members, because the change in your parent's lifestyle can cause upheaval in these relationships.

Many times, what provokes a crisis is that your parent needs another level of care, but will not consider options. If this is the case, there is not a lot you can do; your parent is an adult with the right to make his own decisions. It may take a fall or a medical emergency to get you actively involved in your parent's care.

The Emergency Plan of Action. You can minimize a future health-care crisis by having an emergency plan of action.

- Obtain durable power of attorney for health care and finances forms (see Chapter 23), and discuss the various options with your parent. If your parent is not comfortable having this conversation, back off for a little while and then try again. It is imperative that your parent complete a power of attorney *before* a crisis occurs. Then, if you find yourself making hard decisions, your parent's wishes will be clear to you.

- Obtain the names and numbers of all your parent's attending and consulting physicians.

- Call and introduce yourself to your parent's regular health-care provider(s). Give a copy of the Power of Attorney for Health Care to the doctor and keep a copy for yourself. Keep in mind that your parent's doctor may not be on call when you need him, so always take the power of attorney papers with you, in case you are dealing with a doctor on call who is unfamiliar with your parent's medical condition.

- Obtain photocopies of your parent's Medicare and supplementary insurance (Medigap) identification cards *or* her HMO card (Secure Horizon, Kaiser, Healthnet, etc.). Keep them handy.

- Keep a list of your parent's current medications (such as blood thinners), and make a note of any she is allergic to. If your parent is admitted to an emergency room, the admitting physician will need this list and any other vital information you can provide, such as allergies, chronic medical conditions (for example, diabetes or asthma), past surgeries, and whether your parent has a pacemaker.

- Decide which family member will be able to reach your parent first in case of emergency. This family member must have the above information readily available.

- Make contact with the local nurses registry, or similar organization that provides home health care, and for future reference, ask how readily they can provide assistance. Learn what services are available and how much they cost.

- Familiarize yourself with assisted living or skilled nursing facilities in your parent's area in case your parent is discharged from the hospital and is not allowed to return home.

Christopher and Elena. Christopher was seventy-nine and still a full-time CPA. His sister, Elena, eighty-four, was suffering from end-stage congestive heart failure and had just been released from the hospital. Since she was stubborn about accepting outside help, Christopher was bringing food to Elena's home once a day. He felt guilty that he wasn't doing enough, yet he was also resentful that the entire burden had fallen on his shoulders. When he dropped by at eleven A.M. one day, Elena was still in bed. Her lower extremities were visibly swollen, and she appeared short of breath. She hadn't taken her medication and couldn't remember how to use the oxygen. In addition, she wasn't eating and drinking enough to keep up her strength.

Her brother needed an emergency plan of action. He started by visiting a nursing home. In my office, Christopher appeared at his wits' end. "She's my older sister," he said, "and I never could tell her what to do. She refuses to consider long-term care, and I don't have the energy to fight with her anymore, Stella."

As we spoke, Christopher realized his sister had left him with no real options. I recommended that the next time Elena entered the hospital (which was inevitable, given her shortness of breath and refusal to take medicine), Christopher speak to her physician about issuing a written order stating that Elena required nursing home care and that returning home was not an option. Fearful of the unknown, elderly patients often don't want to leave their home but may experience a secret degree of relief that their physical needs will be professionally cared for.

The next time Elena entered the hospital, Christopher did contact her cardiologist, who agreed that Elena needed twenty-four-hour care. The following week, she was discharged to our care. As her congestive heart failure progressed, her medications were managed to control swelling, and her oxygen was monitored. "I can see from her face that she's not scared like she was at home," Christopher said. His readiness with a plan kept Elena's need for a new level of care from becoming yet another crisis.

II. The Invisible Crisis

An invisible crisis results from a slow loss of physical and/or cognitive function that is ignored until the elder's health and welfare are in a state of marked deterioration. Camouflaged by gradual decline, the resulting crisis is hard to differentiate from what was formerly the patient's normal daily life. For a year or two, your parent may seem to be "doing okay." But there may come a time when you know that your mother is becoming forgetful, that she occasionally misses appointments, and that her housekeeping isn't what it used to be. She may not be sure what the doctor told her about an upcoming procedure. Her life is still filled with family, friends, and daily pleasures, yet you start to wonder if it is safe for her to drive.

All too often, no one pays much attention to small signs that a parent's functioning is slipping. There is denial on both sides. The parent may say, "I'm fine. Nothing has changed, and if it has, I'm dealing with it." Likewise, the adult child often does not want to recognize that Mom's abilities are declining and that she may soon need extra help. Denial comes easily in overscheduled lives—it's easier to look at a parent who has always been self-sufficient and say, "I've got so much on my plate right now. Mom's okay. If it ain't broke, don't fix it."

This is the time to meet as a family and come up with a flexible plan of action for your parent's future, yet few people do. When your parent is relatively healthy, it is awkward to discuss the "what ifs" without feeling rude and intrusive. Discussing your parent's limitations may sound like betrayal. Your siblings may call you an alarmist. Regrettably, your parent may feel affronted and defensive.

If you ignore small warning signs, an invisible crisis deepens until her health, and possibly yours, is at stake. As you intervene more frequently in her day-to-day activities and decisions, neither you nor your parent may want to acknowledge the loss of function or the inability to cope. But gradually, the shortcomings become obvious.

Invisible Crisis Stage One. "Red flags" were identified in Chapter 2. Here is a quick review of conditions that indicate that an invisible crisis may be brewing.

1. Deterioration in personal hygiene
2. Unopened mail, bills not paid, accounts overdrawn
3. Carpets stained with food
4. Trouble remembering recent events
5. Change in eating habits
6. Repeatedly misplacing objects
7. Inability to remember if medications were taken
8. Unexplained bruises
9. Frequent phone calls to you or others
10. Unexplained dents in the car

If your parent shows the signs of physical or cognitive deterioration listed above, it is time to draw up your plan for a gradually higher level of care, either in the home or, if necessary, in a professional setting.

Invisible Crisis Stage Two. Families rarely investigate long-term care for their parent in stage one of an invisible crisis; they seek it in stage two, when the parent's health and safety are endangered and they can no longer deny or cope with the following signs:

1. Musty odor in the house or on clothing
2. Urine-stained carpets
3. Noticeable weight loss or gain
4. Skin tears or open sores

5. Minor car accidents; knocked-off rearview mirrors
6. Repetitive phone calls at odd times
7. Inability to recall how the day was spent
8. Offensive mouth odor
9. Medication bottles too full or too empty
10. "Third and final" notices for phone and electricity payments

At this point, it is difficult to ignore your parent's impairments. Emotions can spin out of control very quickly. Adult children may feel anxiety, fear, anger, and impatience. However, openly discussing shortcomings as they are noticed and having a flexible long-term plan in place can prevent a family meltdown.

III. Advance Long-Term-Care Planning

Paula and Ruth. Paula, a grade-school teacher, breezed into my office one afternoon. "I'm sorry I don't have an appointment," she said, "but my mom insisted I stop by after work and introduce myself. Years ago, she had a dear friend named Jason whom she visited in your nursing home. Mom wasn't sure if you would remember her, but she has never forgotten the care your staff gave Jason."

Now eighty-nine, Paula's mother, Ruth, had suffered from generalized pain for three years. Although pain pills had been effective, she often couldn't remember whether she had taken them, and lately, the medication had been causing constipation. Once when Ruth took a laxative that was too strong, she became so physically weak that her other daughter, Ellie, had to spend a few nights at her house. For the past two weeks, Ruth had become lethargic and was staying in bed all day.

Paula went on, "This morning before I went to work, Mom

called me and announced, 'The time has come for me to move to assisted living at Stella's. You girls have your lives with your husbands, your children, and your careers. I know you worry about me, and honestly I kind of worry myself being here alone.'

"I never thought of Mom getting old, but she did. I told her I'd speak with you today, and she'd like to come with me tomorrow to start taking measurements and making lists for the move. She has always been extremely organized. I hope you have a room for her."

Ruth joined us three weeks later. As I observed the move taking place, I wondered if Paula and Ellie realized the gift their mother had given them. There was no crisis, no panic, no second-guessing, and no sibling misunderstandings. Paula and Ellie never had to convince an angry, unwilling parent that more advanced care was needed.

Planning Gives Control Back to You and Your Parent. As their mother moved to her new home, Paula and Ellie still experienced anxiety and guilt that perhaps they hadn't done enough. But with an organized relocation like Ruth's, emotions are more manageable. The difference between this move and a crisis move is that Ruth was the one who made the plans—her daughters simply carried out her wishes. Talking about and planning for the future well in advance alleviates much of the awkwardness and guilt when the time comes to carry out the plans.

It is important for families to manage their parent's care at home for as long as possible. However, if home care is no longer healthy for either you or your parent, the twenty-four-hour medical care of a good facility is the best option. If long-term care is included in the family plan as a possibility, you can have a manageable, controlled transition that will not escalate into crisis and it will not seem forced on you, should the time come.

When we have control over our day-to-day lives, we find comfort and security. Not having control places us in a victimlike role. Our parents feel exactly the same way. Without a plan, you have to improvise when emergencies strike, and your spur-of-the-moment decisions place your parents in a frightening position. A coordinated plan drawn up in advance by your parents along with you will empower them when they are faced with long-term-care needs. They will not feel victimized or out of control living with decisions they made themselves, and you will have a closer, more supportive relationship as you carry out their express wishes.

11 ✐ LEVELS OF LONG-TERM CARE

When Liz and her husband got home from their two-week cruise, the phone was ringing as they walked through the door. It was Liz's brother, Ted. While they were away, their mother had fractured her hip. "I didn't call you," Ted explained, "because I didn't want to ruin your vacation. Mom is already up and walking in physical therapy. But the hospital discharge planner just called and said Mom needs to be transferred to a skilled rehab center within forty-eight hours. Liz, I have no idea what we're looking for."

When Liz reached me by phone, her voice was trembling. "I don't know what kind of facility Mom needs," she said. "I'm still in shock that she's even in a hospital. The discharge planner gave my brother a list of facilities. Does this mean she needs a nursing home?"

The urgency and bewilderment of Liz's call is a common occurrence. When families call asking for guidance, it doesn't help that the terminology for health-care levels is confusing and irregular. According to Virginia Morris in her book, *How to Care for Aging Parents,* the Health Care Financing Administration has identified forty-four different names for care provided by nursing homes. A recent Met Life survey reveals there are twenty-six names for assisted-living facilities. The choices you have in your community will fall into one of six broad care options.

ASSISTED LIVING

Assisted-living facilities became popular in the 1990s and are now the fastest-growing level of long-term care for seniors in the United States. They bridge the gap between independent living and nursing home care. The many names for assisted living include: board and care, residential care for the elderly, retirement home, adult congregate-living community, and congregate-care retirement. Since each state has its own licensing requirements and regulations to define assisted living, there is considerable variation. This makes choosing assisted living more complicated than choosing nursing homes (which are federally regulated and standardized).

Assisted-living facilities may be small, homelike buildings with as few as six residents, or they can be large, multifloor facilities with hundreds of residents. While some offer no hands-on care, others offer twenty-four-hour care, including help with bathing, dressing, grooming, and medication management. Although the average resident in assisted living requires access to health care twenty-four hours a day, they do not need twenty-four-hour hands-on care. Since these facilities differ widely in their ability to provide continuing care, there is variation in pricing, staffing, services, and admission policies. Some facilities will accept wheelchairs, while others permit only walkers. As residents' physical or cognitive abilities decline, options in assisted living become limited. For example, fire safety regulations often do not allow residents to remain at this level of care if they cannot independently remove themselves from physical danger.

In assisted living, design and furnishings can be more residential than institutional. Decorating rooms with their own furnishings, residents personalize living space as much as possible. Services usually include meals, housekeeping, social activities, transportation, an emergency call system, and help with bathing, dressing, and grooming. Other services, such as medication management, salon hair care, or manicure, are purchased à la carte, as needed by the resident.

Medicare does not pay for assisted living. In many states, Medicaid does not pay for it either. Monthly charges are usually paid out of the resident's own funds, by long-term care insurance, or by the resident's children.

NURSING HOMES (LONG TERM)

A nursing home provides long-term care to residents who are no longer able to take care of their activities of daily living due to functional or cognitive impairments. Staffed around the clock with licensed nursing professionals and other trained personnel, nursing homes provide long-term supportive and custodial care to residents who must be admitted under the care of a physician. Other names you may hear for nursing homes are convalescent homes, nursing centers, care centers, and skilled-nursing facilities. Residents require assistance with bathing, dressing, feeding, transferring in and out of bed, and incontinence care. Most facilities have a mixture of patients with a variety of medical conditions, and typically, the residents are cognitively impaired. According to statistics, more than 40 percent of people over sixty-five will spend at least some time in a nursing home, and more than 50 percent of elders who enter a nursing home will spend the remainder of their lives there. A consequence of being one of the most regulated industries in the United States is the production of cookie-cutter-like facilities. Throughout the United States, nursing homes look like hospitals— right down to the nurses' station, hospital beds, cubicle curtains, and medical record charts.

Confusion About Reimbursement. Most Americans are unaware that Medicare provides very little coverage for nursing home services. The majority of nursing homes provide custodial care, not the rehabilitative care required for Medicare coverage. As a result, nursing home care is paid for on a private, out-of-pocket basis. For low-income residents, each state has a welfare program that will pay for nursing home care for those who qualify. For more information about benefits and eligibility requirements, contact Centers for Medicare and Medicaid Services (CMS). Their website is www.cms.hhs.gov. (Also see Chapter 23.)

REHABILITATIVE-CARE CENTERS (SHORT TERM)

Rehab-care centers are for short-term residents who are recovering from an injury or illness, most commonly a fracture or a stroke. Most rehab units consist of a designated number of beds within a hospital or a skilled-nursing facility. Residents no longer need the acute services of a hospital but still require skilled rehabilitative care. This typically means in-patient physical, occupational, or speech therapy, as well as monitoring by licensed nurses for IV therapy, tube feeding, and sterile dressings for bed sores and for postsurgery wounds.

The Medicare handbook leads you to believe your parent is entitled to one hundred days of Medicare coverage for rehabilitation care. In fact, stringent guidelines must be met:

1. Your parent must have spent at least three consecutive nights in the hospital. However, a hospital stay resulting in nursing home care does not automatically qualify your parent for Medicare-paid rehabilitation. This is a common misunderstanding.

2. Your parent must need skilled care related to the condition for which she was treated in the hospital, and it must be an illness or injury she can demonstrably recover from in a reasonable amount of time.

3. Your parent must receive the rehab services in a Medicare-certified facility within thirty days of his hospital discharge.

4. Your parent's doctor must certify the need for skilled nursing or skilled rehab care.

If your parent meets these guidelines, Medicare will pay for a limited period of time. The first twenty days will be 100 percent covered. Should coverage continue to the twenty-first day, Medicare will pay all but a daily copayment for a maximum of one hundred days. This daily copay is $119 in 2006 and will be adjusted annually. (Your parent's Medigap or Medicaid will cover the copayment. See Chapter 23 for the importance of supplemental insurance.) After day one hundred, there is no coverage; when Medicare stops, so does the supplemental insurance. The majority of Medicare coverage lasts approximately twenty days.

If your parent does not qualify for Medicare, private funds will have to be used. If private funds are not available, low-income residents may be eligible for Medicaid programs, which vary from state to state. (Again, see Chapter 23.) If your parent belongs to an HMO, options for rehabilitative services will be limited to HMO-contracted facilities only.

Introduce Yourself to the Hospital Discharge Planner. The discharge planner (sometimes called the social worker) at the hospital is responsible for discharging patients in a timely manner, so as not to incur unnecessary financial consequences for the hospital. Since every patient is assigned a social worker upon admission, find out who has been assigned to your parent and start communicating with her. The social worker can tell you when the discharge is likely to occur and whether your parent is a candidate for Medicare-paid rehab services or relocation to a nursing home for custodial care. The earlier you establish a relationship with the discharge planner, the less surprised you'll be when you are given a discharge date.

If your parent qualifies for rehab, ask if there is a rehab unit within the hospital and if a bed is available. If so, make this your first choice. Staying within the same hospital grounds will be easier on your parent. If the hospital does not have a rehab unit or an available bed, ask the social worker for the name of facilities she feels comfortable recommending in the area. While this is a good place to start, be aware that many social workers prefer to work with just one or two nursing homes or rehab centers. It is still a good idea to ask your parent's physician and your friends for recommendations, and to tap into good old-fashioned word of mouth for the names of good places close to your home.

SPECIAL-CARE UNITS

A special care unit can be either a free-standing facility, or a unit within an assisted-living facility or nursing home. These units focus on the care of residents with specific medical conditions such as Alzheimer's. Now becoming more commonplace, special care units arose from the need for more specialized care not routinely available in nursing homes. The staff has been specially trained to deal with dementia, and the units have a physical design that promotes safe mobility. For the wandering resident, these units provide as much as possible an environment free of physical and chemical restraint. Special care units have a fire safety clearance that allows doors to remain locked, so that a wandering patient will be unable to exit the facility. Safety is maximized, yet the resident is able to walk around at will. Door alarms, outside fencing, and other security systems protect the environment for the resident. There is no Medicare provision for special care units.

CONTINUING-CARE RETIREMENT COMMUNITY

Continuing-care retirement communities (CCRCs), sometimes also called life care communities, combine three levels of care: independent living, assisted living, and nursing home—all on a single campus. These communities are designed using the aging-in-place theory; that is, your parent can move in as an active member of society and remain for the rest of her life. She may have to transfer to a different building when more care is needed, but the grounds and management remain the same. Continuing-care retirement communities provide rooms or apartments, meals, and health care. They may also provide activities such as trips, social programs, religious

115

services, and exercise classes. The drawback is that CCRCs can be expensive. Often, there is a sizable entrance fee in addition to monthly maintenance fees. Religious or other nonprofit organizations sponsor most CCRCs.

HOSPICE CARE

Hospice remains a largely misunderstood and underutilized service in health care for those with limited life expectancy. As a philosophy of care, hospice focuses on the importance of dignity and freedom from pain at life's end. It emphasizes palliative management of symptoms, that is, compassionate care rather than aggressive cure-oriented intervention. In the past, hospice care was generally provided in the home, but more and more it is available in assisted-living facilities and nursing homes as well. Traditionally, hospice care focused on cancer, but now it also covers patients with end-stage diseases such as Alzheimer's, congestive heart failure, and renal failure. A partnership between family, hospice personnel, and nursing home or assisted-living facility can significantly improve end-of-life care.

The Medicare hospice benefit will supply an interdisciplinary team skilled in pain management, symptom control, and bereavement assistance. In addition, it will pay for durable medical equipment, such as oxygen equipment, walkers, and wheelchairs, as well as medicines ordered by the hospice team. A copayment of $5 or less per drug may apply. A physician must certify that the patient has six months or less to live. This federally required certification has caused confusion to families who are considering hospice. However, the duration of hospice care can be reviewed and extended indefinitely. If your parent is faced with limited life expectancy, hospice offers active care to meet the physical, psychological, and spiritual needs of both the patient and the family.

The Future of Long-Term Care

Our current level of skilled-nursing health care for the aged has not worked. Historically, government regulators have focused on health and safety. But what about satisfaction, service, and quality of life? These are equally important in a place you plan to call home. Since no one wants to live in a highly restricted environment, nursing homes are declining in popularity while assisted-living and continuing-care facilities are on the rise.

In the coming years, the baby boomer generation will enter long-term care in unprecedented numbers. Born between 1946 and 1964, the boomers have had a profound effect on public policy so far at every stage of their life. As the next generation to require nursing home services, boomers are faced with the challenge of redefining long-term care. We need a social revolution—one that will solve the coming long-term-care crisis that threatens to break the backbone of our health-care system. The current lack of vision demands the development of systems and facilities unique to this generation. Will boomers accept the standard nursing homes of today? I hope not. We need to reawaken the political clout used so well forty years ago and force the long-term-care profession into a consumer-oriented, user-friendly, service-driven industry. The choice is ours.

12 ✐ WHERE DO YOU START?

Answering my office phone late one Friday afternoon, I heard a concerned woman say, "My mom needs a nursing home, but there are so many distressing stories about them. How do I find the right one?"

"How did you hear about us?" I asked.

She replied, "Several years ago, you took care of my best friend's mother, and she said you would help me."

How do you find a quality nursing home or an assisted-living facility for your parent? The following are eight suggestions I've shared with families to help them begin their search:

> 1. Word-of-mouth recommendations are an excellent place to start; there is no source more reliable than someone you know and trust. In the past, women of my generation had lunch and discussed how to locate the right orthodontist for their children. Today, the same

women are networking to locate the best long-term-care facility for their parents. If the name of a particular facility is mentioned again and again, be sure to file it away for future reference.

2. The local senior center in your area can provide a list of nursing homes within a comfortable radius of your neighborhood. Ask to speak with the social service specialist.

3. Religious social service organizations, such as Jewish Family Services or Catholic Charities, can also serve as a good point of reference.

4. Your family doctor, hospital social worker, and clergy may provide you with good leads as well. Be sure to ask if they have personally visited the nursing home, or if they are sharing someone else's experience with you. Recommendations from firsthand knowledge will be the most dependable.

5. Organizations such as Alzheimer's Association, Parkinson's Association, or National Stroke Association will have a list of facilities in your area. Each of these illnesses has special requirements, and it is important to admit your parent to a facility equipped to meet his type and level of care.

6. Geriatric-care managers play a new role in the field in geriatrics. As licensed social workers or registered nurses, they come to your home, assess the situation, and recommend appropriate in-home services or a more advanced level of care, if necessary. Contact the National Association of Professional Geriatric Care Managers.

7. Your local Area Agency on Aging will give you a list of licensed facilities in your area as well as the phone number for the nearest location of the Office of the Long-Term Care Ombudsman. As state advocates for elderly residents, ombudsmen routinely visit assisted living facilities and nursing homes; consequently, they are knowledgeable about the features and the quality of care each facility offers. Contact Eldercare Locator at 800-677-1116.

8. The Internet can be a useful tool. However, facility websites may be no more than advertisements, and government-posted inspection reports are frequently out-of-date, difficult to understand, and open to misinterpretation. Consider the Internet for general information only.

Nolan. A gentleman I didn't recognize was walking up and down the hall of our care facility. "Can I help you?" I asked.

Introducing himself as Nolan, he showed me his book on how to choose a nursing home. "This author recommends that I come in unannounced," he said, "but now that I'm here, I'm not sure what to do next. Just looking into people's rooms isn't getting me anywhere."

On the way to my office, Nolan explained that his ninety-two-year-old mother had been self-sufficient until the previous week, when she had fallen and hit her head. Admitted to the hospital for tests, she was still quite weak. "They say she'll be discharged the day after tomorrow and that she needs nursing home care," he continued. "Even though my brother has visited three nursing homes already, I'd like to have an informed conversation with him, so I'm doing some research of my own. This book says to be sure to ask about staffing ratios and inspection reports." He paused. "I have no idea what they're talking about."

Can You Rely on Inspection Reports?

Inspection reports for every nursing home in the United States are available on the Internet. Go to medicare.gov and click on "Nursing Home Compare." In these reports you will find survey results, deficiency patterns, staffing information, number of beds, type of ownership, and whether the facility participates in Medicare, Medicaid, or both.

Staffing Reports. Since facilities are generally surveyed by the Department of Healthcare Services every twelve to fifteen months, information you find can be out-of-date. Although data posted on the Internet may prove valuable, you cannot assess resident care and quality-of-life issues from a government graph. More important is how long the current administrator and director of nurses have been responsible for the facility—frequent turnover of these positions will have a great impact on quality of care. A personal visit continues to be your best bet in finding a quality care facility because it allows you to observe the staff, *and the staff is the most important element in the success of a nursing home.*

Staff-to-resident ratio is one indicator of the quality of care your parent will receive. An acceptable ratio of nurse's aides to residents would be as follows:

Day Shift	one nurse's aide to six residents
Evening Shift	one nurse's aide to ten residents
Night Shift	one nurse's aide to fourteen residents

This ratio should be maintained seven days a week.

Ask if the licensed nurses and nurse's aides are full-time employees or if the facility works with nursing registries (temporary agencies). If the facility is staffed with registry nurses, it will be unable to offer the same level of care as one that hires, monitors, and educates its own staff.

The Inspection Report

Pamphlets advising consumers how to choose a nursing home often give state inspection reports a lot of credibility. However, these reports do not necessarily portray the facilities accurately. When I look up nursing homes in Los Angeles on the Internet, it makes me uneasy to see respectable ratings for facilities that I personally know are undergoing difficulties. Although survey findings may be useful to establish a record of repeated violations, they do not begin to tell the full story. Facilities that look good on paper may not be delivering quality care. The inspectors' interpretation of regulations can be subjective and inconsistent. Survey teams, short staffed due to poor government funding, are responsible for completing a sea of paperwork when their time could be better spent evaluating actual hands-on care given to patients.

Certainly, government inspections have helped to improve long-term care, for example, by exposing high incidences of bedsores, frequent falls, and overuse of physical and chemical restraints. Over time, however, the surveys have become more of a punitive instrument, imposing stiff monetary fines for violating regulations, but doing little to improve patient care. Often, facilities simply add more staff whose sole responsibility is to improve the paperwork, not the quality of care.

If you like what you've learned about a facility, but you have read a survey report and feel uncomfortable about certain deficiencies, ask the administrator for an explanation. If she is open and able to explain your findings, this may still be a desirable facility.

Making the Phone Calls. Once you have developed a list of facilities, use the phone to request information regarding facility size and location. The cost should be established before visiting the premises. Are there additional fees? Is there a bed available? If your parent has special needs, can the facility accommodate him? If it is a nursing home, is it certified for Medicare and Medicaid funds? Is there a religious affiliation?

From the first hello, whether you notice it or not, the facility is already making an impression on you. Ask yourself these questions: How did you feel about the call? Was the staff member you spoke to friendly and attentive? If she couldn't answer your questions, did she transfer you to someone who could? Did you feel as if you wanted to know more about the facility? If not, proceed down your list.

When you have narrowed your choices to three or four facilities, plan to visit each one, preferably during the lunch hour. Although visiting during lunch will limit you to one facility per day, it will provide you with useful information. For example, by noon, residents should be up and dressed, and their rooms neat and orderly. The meal being served should look fresh, appetizing, and nutritious. This is a good opportunity to observe the staff. Are they interacting with the residents, or are they speaking mainly to each other?

The Walk-Through and the Inquiry Process. Two things are essential in determining if the care facility is best for your parent:

1. A physical walk-through with a professional staff member.
2. A formal, in-depth meeting, which I call the "inquiry process" (see Chapter 15). I strongly recommend that you meet with the administrator or with the director of nurses.

You will find questionnaires in books and on the Internet to help choose a facility. Most of them consist of items to be checked yes or no to keep track of and narrow your choices. If you take one of these checklists with you on your visit, do not let it distract you from the two essentials above. Remember, your parent's individual needs and personality are not on the checklist.

Making Your Decision. Rank the facilities you have visited in the order of your preference. If time permits, revisit your first and second choices, this time choosing another time of day, perhaps during activities, to give you a more complete "feel" for the surroundings. Observe the staff one more time, bearing in mind it is the staff, the hands-on caregivers, who will determine your parent's well-being in her new home.

Anne, seventy-six, sank gratefully into the chair
across from me, exhausted from her search for a
facility. Before I could say hello, she sighed, "I'm so
tired and confused. I'm not sure where my husband
needs to be. For three years, I've taken care of him at
home, and we've been fine," she continued. "Then last
Saturday morning, I couldn't wake him up. I got scared
and called 911. He's been in the hospital for five days
now, and I need to find a place for him by tomorrow.
The doctor says I can't take care of him at home any
longer.

"So the discharge planner at the hospital gave me
this list of facilities," she went on. "The first one I saw
was a small six-bed house. The next was a large, two-
story hotel-type place that felt too big. The third looked
like a hospital. I know he doesn't need a hospital, but
what am I looking for?"

"It can get complicated, Anne," I confirmed. "The

two most common levels of care are assisted living and nursing homes. Because of federal regulations, all nursing homes resemble hospitals. Assisted-living facilities look more homelike."

Assisted Living

Although the generic name is "assisted living," these facilities are known variously throughout the country as board and care, residential care for the elderly, retirement home, adult congregate-living community, congregate-care retirement, and many other names. In the United States, assisted living is the fastest-growing type of senior housing. Unlike federally regulated nursing homes, assisted-living facilities are regulated by individual states; therefore, there is enormous variety across the country, ranging from small board-and-care cottages to elaborate hotels. Interestingly, in some states, schools have been converted into assisted-living facilities, reflecting the demographic changes in America!

The goal of assisted living is to assist with basic personal needs, such as bathing, dressing, and grooming, while keeping the resident active and engaged in the community. Assisted living fosters independence, personal dignity, and privacy. In many facilities, transportation to movies, shopping, or other outings may be available. Assisted living may also offer partial health care, such as "medication management" (taking the correct pills on time).

Fire safety regulations require that residents in assisted living be physically and mentally able to get themselves out of danger in case of emergencies such as earthquake or fire. Increasingly, however, there is a blurring of definitions as to how these regulations are enforced. For example, fire regulations are being more loosely interpreted to allow mentally competent residents with physical restrictions to stay in assisted living. It is important to be aware of your parent's abilities regarding emergency issues.

While assisted-living facilities do not offer comprehensive twenty-four-hour medical and nursing care, they generally do provide the following:

1. Assistance with bathing, dressing, grooming, and personal hygiene
2. Twenty-four-hour supervision
3. Three meals a day
4. Medication management
5. Assistance with toileting and incontinence issues
6. Housekeeping and laundry
7. Social activities, such as ceramics and exercise classes, lectures, shopping, and outings to local theater
8. Emergency call system (In the bathroom and by the bed, a call cord is required to notify staff in case of emergency)

Cost Is a Consideration

Since Medicare does not pay for assisted living, and Medicaid pays very little, virtually all expenses are out-of-pocket for families or residents. Currently fees range from $2,000 to $8,000 a month. Services may be covered by one all-inclusive monthly rate, or they may be à la carte based on individual needs. When searching for a facility, it is important to ask what that monthly fee includes, as well as what it does not include. Look carefully at elaborate fee structures, as they can add hundreds, even thousands to the monthly bill. Are there different charges for different levels of care? Is a deposit required? What are the total monthly costs?

Where Does Your Family Member Belong?

As an introduction to community living, assisted living is preferred because of the homelike atmosphere. Considering that moving a parent out of her home will probably cause guilt and misgivings, the transition is easier and less threatening for both of you.

As I sat and talked with Anne, it became clear to me that her husband was an assisted-living candidate—he could get out of a chair unassisted and his physical needs were well within the parameters of assisted-living care. Once we had determined his status, Anne wanted to revisit the other assisted-living facilities she had seen. "What should I look for?" she asked.

"Fortunately, a walk-through in assisted living is less complicated than a walk-through in a nursing home," I told Anne. "Here is a guide to help you evaluate the facilities":

1. Do the residents have the same level of abilities or disabilities that your family member has? In some facilities, the majority of residents may be in advanced stages of dementia. In others, they may be attending lectures on current events and participating in exercise classes. Which facility would be best for your parent?
2. Does the facility have a homelike environment? Would you be comfortable visiting?
3. Will the facility offer a measure of privacy and independence for your parent?
4. Is there a smoking policy?
5. Are the activities in places that are accessible if your parent uses a walker?
6. Watch residents engaged in an activity. Are they enjoying themselves? Are they socializing? Is there interaction between the activities director and the residents?

7. Is the facility too large or small for your parent? Just as some teenagers prefer a large or small college, your parent may have a preference as well.

8. Is there an emergency call cord by the bedside and in the bathroom?

9. Does the staff greet or acknowledge you as you walk by?

10. Look at staff-resident interaction; does the staff treat residents with respect and dignity?

11. Is there an unpleasant odor? Although odor should not be an issue in assisted living, it can be a red flag that there are housekeeping and personal-care problems.

12. Does the food look appetizing? Do residents seem to enjoy their meals? Would you be allowed to sample a meal?

13. Does the facility have a van to transport your parent to shopping, the theater, or to his doctor's office?

14. Is the facility licensed? If not, it means the care is not being monitored by the state, and this puts an added responsibility on the family.

15. Ask who is responsible for the health care of your parent during a medical emergency. For example, if your parent needed medical attention during the night, who would arrange it?

Be Aware of Your Parent's Needs

As your parent ages in place at the assisted-living facility, be aware that the status of his mental and physical health will change. When you notice his physical needs increasing, or his cognitive abilities diminishing, it may be time to reassess whether the facility is still offering the appropriate level of care. If you find that your parent is not taking his medicine, that his clothing is soiled, that he is losing weight, or that his behavior is changing, speak with the administrator and voice your concerns. Ask if the facility can continue to safely and successfully accommodate your parent as his health and medical needs increase. If the administrator says yes, but your parent continues to lose weight, or fails to take his medications, begin looking into nursing home options before a crisis develops. You do not want a call from the facility saying, "We can no longer take care of your parent." Nor do you want your parent to remain in a level of care that is inappropriate for his needs.

Time to Relocate Once More

Most families are relieved to find a homelike assisted-living facility where their parent is safe and socially engaged. For a time, it can be the ideal situation. You may think, Dad can just remain here. He'll never need a nursing home. However, assisted living should not be considered an alternative to nursing home care. As residents become more frail and forgetful, the assisted-living environment can become dangerous to their health and safety. The average length of residence in assisted living is three years. In my experience, the most common reason for discharge is the need for a nursing home. This surprises many families who do not expect another relocation. Just as they become accustomed to assisted living, it is time to educate themselves about nursing home care.

Society has a bias against nursing homes, but professionally run, caring homes do exist. To locate them, you must become a sophisticated, knowledgeable consumer. The next chapters are an essential guide to finding a high-quality, professional nursing home that will care for your parent and be helpful and supportive to your family.

14 🐚 A WALK THROUGH
A NURSING HOME

"I've dreaded this day all my life."
"I didn't sleep last night thinking about today."
*"I was afraid of the noises, the smells, and the people I
would see."*
"My sister asked me to take a look. She couldn't face it."

These are thoughts families have shared with me in
their search for nursing home care. Most were in crisis.
The discharge planner at the hospital may have given
them only twenty-four hours' notice to find a care center. Too late, families discover that it takes time to find a
quality facility that offers personalized medical care and
homelike atmosphere.

If you are not prepared, a nursing home can be in-
timidating. Many long-term-care guides recommend
that you walk through a facility without announcing
yourself to determine how it feels to you. If you are
experienced and comfortable in a long-term-care set-

ting, this may be helpful. However, if you are just beginning your search, a good administrator or director of nurses can guide you through this unknown territory. Because emotions will run high during the search for an appropriate facility, you might consider bringing a friend or family member with you, perhaps someone with long-term-care experience.

A Different World

Many years ago, Pam came to see me about placing her seventy-six-year-old mother in the nursing home. She was an anxious daughter and, at the time, I was a novice in my first year working in a long-term-care facility. Since those days, my greatest teachers have been my residents and their families. The knowledge I have today, I owe to them. But back then, I had a lot to learn. After I asked Pam a few questions, I took her on a tour. As we walked into the activity room, I noticed her face was ashen. "Are you okay?" I asked her.

"Not really. Can we go back to your office?" Pam replied weakly.

"I'm sorry," she sighed as she sat down, "but I feel light-headed. The sea of wheelchairs and white-haired ladies was too much for me. I can't picture my mother here." Unable to visualize what the tour would involve, Pam had been overwhelmed, and I was not much help. I determined that in the future I would prepare families more carefully for their introduction to long-term care.

Preconceived Notions

"I hope my relatives don't think I'm selfish looking into long-term care for my mom, but I work such long hours," said Caroline, a TV producer, as we walked toward my office. "This is the first nursing home I've ever been in," she said, looking around. "I have heard such horror stories. My friends tell me these places are unpleasant, understaffed, and uncaring. At least yours doesn't smell of urine or disinfectant." She spoke very quickly, as if certain things needed to be said up front.

"Our staff works hard to have an odor-free facility," I acknowledged. "It requires constant vigilance. Caroline, let me tell you a little bit about who we are, and then if we sound like an appropriate level of care for your mother, we'll go on a tour." For almost an hour, Caroline and I talked. My goal was to paint a picture with words of what we would be seeing on our walk through the nursing home. As we started down the corridor, Caroline asked, "Can I speak to the patients?"

"They will love the interaction," I replied. Caroline talked and joked with some of the residents, and I introduced her to other family members who were visiting.

As we returned to the office, she said, "I had dreaded this visit so much, and now it's done. It was much easier than I thought it would be." Facing her fear by discussing anxieties and preconceived notions before touring the nursing home allowed Caroline to feel empowered. Observing your parent's decline is not easy. However, taking control of this new phase in your parent's life can give you a measure of calm and strength.

Why Is the Walk-Through Frightening?

What makes touring a nursing home so difficult? Many things. When there are serious time constraints, you must literally learn as you go. You may feel pressure to make a fast decision. Everything is new and not necessarily pleasant. Because a nursing home may be thought of as "a place you go to die," the decision to place a family member is often accompanied by guilt and remorse. Further, the elderly may be perceived as unattractive, frail, depressed, and obsolete. Since society has done a good job convincing us that this is true, seeing large numbers of ailing seniors in one place can be unsettling.

Our generation struggles with aging issues. Antiaging creams, Botox, liposuction, and countless plastic surgery procedures confirm that we are working way too hard on remaining forever young. Many adults I talk to seem convinced that advanced age and weakened health will not affect them personally. As Lillian, a tanned, chic woman in her seventies who was visiting her mother joked with me, "Stella, I simply do not plan on getting old."

When I began my career in long-term care, I was twenty-two years old. At that time, the advanced age of my residents did not bother me. On the contrary, their continual delight in my youth boosted my self-esteem. Thirty-seven years later, however, the age of my residents has a different effect on me. My residents have gray hair; I have gray hair. They experience aches and pains that I can relate to now. And when I see their adult children anxious and fearful of making the wrong decision, I remember my uncertainty when taking care of my own father and mother.

Each Facility Has a Different Personality

Once you visit three or four facilities, you will discover that each has its own personality. Years ago, as director of patient care services for a large corporation, I was responsible for ensuring quality nursing care in eight long-term-care facilities on the west side of Los Angeles. I made weekly visits to meet with each administrator and director of nurses. As soon as I entered the front door, I could "feel" the personality of the facility. If the administrator and the director of nurses were organized, worked well together, and appreciated their staff, I felt a calm as I entered. If they did not communicate well and were not well organized, I could feel unrest. "It does not take long to become a sophisticated consumer of long-term care," I tell families who seek advice. "Trust your inner sense. As you walk into any long-term-care facility, your initial feeling should be one of comfort and caring."

The Walk-Through

This is not the time for a detailed checklist. As the name implies, the walk-through is a brief tour to get a feel for the facility. Here are some factors to consider:

Greetings. Are you greeted as you enter the facility? There are reasons why this is significant. First, this is the resident's home; we all greet company as they enter our home to indicate they are welcome. Second, it is important for the staff to know who is entering the building.

Acknowledgment and Morale. As you walk down the halls, do the staff members smile and acknowledge you? Do you get a sense of staff morale? High morale is a benchmark of quality care.

Odor. Does an odor of stale urine permeate the building? Keep in mind that if a nurse has just finished changing a resident and has carried soiled clothing to the designated bin in the hallway, there will be a temporary odor that should dissipate in five to ten minutes. But if the odor of urine is persistent, poor housekeeping or poor nursing care may be responsible. Even more offensive than unpleasant odor is the attempt to cover it up with strong antiseptic air fresheners.

Grooming. Are residents up and dressed appropriately for the time of day and the season? Is their hair combed? Are the men shaved and groomed? Are they wearing shoes and socks?

Kindness. Does the staff interact kindly with the residents, addressing them by name, or do they converse as if the residents were not present? Do they speak in demeaning baby talk?

Homelike Atmosphere. Nursing homes are federally regulated to "look like a hospital" with hospital beds, cubicle curtains, and nursing stations. Facilities do, however, have control over atmosphere. Does the nursing home have a homelike feel? Are there family pictures on the residents' walls and nightstands, and afghans or comforters on the beds? Are families allowed to bring in favorite chairs or dressers? Is there a pleasant, central gathering area?

Call Bells. When residents ring for help, the call panel at the nurses' station lights up and sounds an alarm to signal the room number. If the alarm persists, the staff is not responding in a timely manner. Ask the person giving the tour how long it should be before a nurse's aide attends to the resident. An acceptable answer is "less than five minutes."

Pace. Does the staff appear rushed or tense, as if they have too much to do? The work rhythm of the staff should appear calm and steady.

Privacy. If you are touring the facility in the morning—a bathing and dressing period—are residents given privacy? For example, the cubicle curtain should be drawn around the resident's bed during morning care. The same applies in the evening, when residents are changed into nightclothes. Since residents frequently share rooms in nursing homes, privacy curtains help to preserve their dignity. Prior to entering a resident's room, do staff members stop and knock on the doors?

Lunch. A good time to tour a facility is during the noon meal. By this time, everyone should be up and dressed. Their rooms should be organized and neat. As you walk through the dining room, does the food look and smell appetizing? Can you sample the meal being served? Are most of the residents eating in the dining room rather than in their rooms? Do they appear to be enjoying their meal? Are they being assisted? Are any sitting in front of untouched meal trays?

The Menu. Ask to see the posted menu for the week. Is the meal scheduled for the day being served?

Activities. Activity calendars are usually prominently posted for residents and families. Read the current week's activities. Do they cover a broad range of interests such as music, exercise, and current-events classes? If your tour doesn't include the activity area, ask to see it. If a class is scheduled, is it currently in progress? Is it well attended? Do residents seem busy and involved?

The Activities Director. If possible, meet the activities director. Ask how long she has held the position. Since your parent may spend several hours a day with this person, does she seem approachable?

A First-Name Basis. My experience has been that the majority of residents choose to be called by their first name or a nickname they have used all their lives. Ask your parent, or use your best judgment as to what she would like to be called. During the tour, observe the staff's interactions with the residents. If you are uncomfortable hearing them use terms like "Sweetie" or "Baby" in speaking with a resident, let your tour guide know. Your input makes a difference.

How Do You Feel About Your Walk-Through?

Did you get a sense that this was a safe, caring environment where your parent would be well cared for? Is it a place you would be comfortable visiting? Based on the walk-through, would you like to continue on to the more formal inquiry, the fact-finding portion of the facility interview? (See Chapter 15.) The inquiry is a longer, more in-depth analysis of your parent, her needs, and the facility's philosophy of care. Because of the often urgent nature of a nursing home move, the walk-through and the inquiry frequently take place during the same visit. The inquiry should be with either the facility administrator or the director of nursing, but preferably the administrator, because as decision maker for the entire facility, she will have invaluable input.

15 · THE INQUIRY WITH THE FACILITY ADMINISTRATOR
Is This the Right Facility for Your Parent?

"This is the fourth nursing home I've seen today," said Mike, visibly frustrated. "Mom will be discharged from the hospital tomorrow morning, and I'm no better off now than I was when I started. I'm about at the end of my rope, but this is one of the most important decisions I will ever make for her."

"Mike," I replied, "you may feel drained from visiting several facilities, but you will be surprised how much you have learned. You will have better questions to ask me, and your sense of what feels right about a facility will be sharper."

Visiting facilities can be tiring and depressing, but it is time well spent. You will be better prepared for the inquiry, a meeting during which you sit down and discuss your parent with the administrator. An experienced, knowledgeable administrator will help you draw an accurate picture of your parent and her current daily needs regarding physical impairments, cognitive functioning, behavioral problems, safety concerns, and sociability issues. Together, you will determine if the facility can offer the appropriate level of care for your parent and support your needs as a family caregiver as well. Following are questions an administrator should include in her meeting with you:

What are your parent's current diagnoses?

What medications does she take?

Does she require medication management?

Has she ever hidden her medications instead of taking them?

Does your mother become frightened or angry when helped with bathing or dressing?

Can she get in and out of a chair unassisted?

Does she use a walker or a cane?

Has she fallen recently? How often in the past three months?

Does she wander throughout the house during the day? At night?

Has she ever wandered away from home?

How does your parent spend her day?

How is her short-term memory? Can she remember what she had for breakfast?

Can she tell you how she spent the day yesterday?

How is her long-term memory?

Are there particular things that agitate her?

What communication strategies work best?

Is she hard of hearing?

Does she have any visual impairment?

Has she shown signs of incontinence?

Does your parent sleep through the night?

Is her appetite good? Does she require extra time to eat?

Has she lost weight in the past six months?

A Lesson in Asking the Right Questions

Many years ago, Kate and I spent forty minutes discussing her mother's condition before she went on the formal tour of our assisted living. At seventy-eight, Kate's mother, Iris, lived at home and had a paid caregiver every day from seven A.M. to seven P.M. The other twelve hours, Kate herself was on duty, but the responsibility was taking a toll on her. "Even with medication, my blood pressure is out of sight. My doctor says if I don't do something soon, I'll end up flat on my back."

According to Kate, her mother used a walker, could get in and out of a chair unassisted, and was "more continent than not." Although her short-term memory was beginning to be a problem, she merely repeated herself now and then. It appeared Iris would qualify for assisted living.

The following day, Kate brought Iris to see our facility. As I walked out to greet them, Kate was unsuccessfully attempting to maneuver her mother out of the backseat of the car. Since Iris appeared unsteady on her feet, we brought a wheelchair for her. As we toured the rooms, Iris took my hand and said, "I'm so happy to see you again; we had such a lovely lunch last week." I asked Kate if she thought I reminded her mother of someone. "Not that I know of," Kate answered. "Mom hasn't been out of the house for years."

Later, it became apparent Iris had soiled her clothing. When the staff tried to help her, she insisted she was fine and began to remove her clothing in the hallway.

This was not the woman Kate and I had talked about. It was evident Iris would require a different plan of care from the one we had been contemplating. As administrator, it is my responsibility to help families recognize their denial and to pinpoint the parent's actual medical and emotional needs.

Your Responsibility at the Inquiry

A good inquiry establishes a solid foundation for communication. There are otherwise excellent books on long-term care that advise you to "be discreet" about your parent's true condition, for fear a facility will turn your parent away. I disagree with this thinking. As caregiver, your responsibility is to describe your parent's current needs as clearly and completely as you can. An administrator needs to know your parent's health and social needs *as of this meeting*. Any detail you share will help determine the correct level of care. For example, families have been forthright enough to disclose the following with me:

"Mom is not going to like any food you serve her. I've tried everything."

"Dad will not be happy wherever he is. He's not happy at home, and he probably won't be happy here."

"Mom can be difficult during her bath. I always dread the day I have to help the caregiver."

Difficult Behavior Calls for a Special Plan

When families confide problems, the facility is able to design an individualized plan of care. Not divulging behavioral problems can lead to inappropriate placement, and you may find yourself looking at facilities again, starting the whole process over.

Sarah. In the course of an interview, Sarah mentioned that her mother had "vocalization problems." Curious about the terminology, I asked if this meant yelling and hollering, and Sarah reluctantly confirmed my suspicions. When I asked how many times a day, Sarah stammered, "Well, not many..."

Pursuing the subject, I asked "Sarah, in a twenty-four-hour period, how often does your mother call out or holler?"

Hesitating, Sarah finally replied, "about half the day." Sarah's mother will need a special plan of care.

Julie. Before Julie even introduced herself on the phone, she stated up front, "My father bites, scratches, and screams anytime you touch him, so before I come in to see the facility, I need to know if you can take care of him."

When Julie arrived at my office an hour later, I could see scratches on her face and arms. "Dad's been doing this to me and his caregivers for weeks," she explained. "Then yesterday, he slipped out of his chair and broke his leg. When we went to the emergency room, the doctor just put a brace on it, told me he's not a candidate for surgery, and sent us home." Julie paused to regain her composure. "Now he's totally unmanageable. He screams any time we try to move him or change his diaper. The pain medication isn't helping at all." She leaned back in the chair. "I've had it," she sobbed.

By the time Julie's father arrived at our nursing home, we had consulted with his physician and had devised a personalized plan of care. We implemented a new strategy for pain management along with a small dose of antianxiety medication. While he settled in, the staff was made aware of possible physical outbursts. The better the communication at the inquiry, the better the chances of a successful long-term-care experience.

Wandering

Once, after unknowingly admitting a resident who wandered, I was belatedly informed by her daughter, "Well, Mom never wandered at home because Dad put special locks on all the doors. We didn't think she'd do it here." The wandering resident needs a specifically planned and protected environment where he can pace without being a danger to himself. If your parent wanders, make sure the facility you choose offers this level of care.

Special Eating Patterns

Libby, an eighty-nine-year-old resident, had no problem feeding herself, but it could take her over an hour to finish her meal. Since the staff had been made aware of her eating pattern, they knew not to rush her or to mistakenly clear her tray when she put her fork down to rest. If your parent needs assistance with meals or if it takes her more than forty-five minutes to finish eating, ask the administrator if the staff has this kind of time to feed your parent. Some families arrange to visit during meals to help with feeding while others hire private companions to assist with lunch or dinner.

Levels of Sociability

Before her health needs changed, was your parent a social person who enjoyed company? There is a good chance that a previously social person will enjoy getting involved again. The activities director will review the calendar with the resident and invite her to attend specific daily activities.

If, on the other hand, your parent has preferred to keep to herself most of her life, then our staff will approach her more slowly. Sometimes it is a success just to get a resident to the activity room for coffee and cookies. As much as possible, the facility should try to accommodate individual levels of sociability.

Your Parent Then; Your Parent Now

"Mom was so intelligent," said Wendy. "Everyone came to her for advice. I was always proud to say that beautiful lady was my mother."

"Dad treated everyone fair and square," said Burt. "You should have known him when he was the foreman of a large printing shop. All his printers respected him. He's the reason I succeeded in my own business."

Because it can feel like betrayal explaining that a parent has behavioral problems, families frequently start the conversation by telling me their parent's past strengths to let me know I will be caring for someone special. "I'm sorry I never knew the person you are describing," I respond, "but with your help, I will learn who your parent is now. This is important to me and the staff."

When I observe a family's anguish as they describe their parent's difficult behavior, I want to stop the conversation, lean forward, and say, "My dad was like that, too," or "My mom's behavior was also pretty undignified at times. Please don't worry about shocking me."

It's hard to relate that your father must be fed, or that he takes food out of his mouth partially chewed, unsure what to do next. It's not easy to share that your mother is experiencing frequent bowel and bladder issues. If your parent needs help with dressing, eating, and toileting, volunteer this information. If he is a wanderer, suffers from anxiety, refuses to bathe, or is verbally and/or physically abusive, say so. These things can be dealt with, but safeguards must be put in place so the staff can be prepared.

How Do You Feel About Your Visit?

Problem solving for your parent's care and comfort begins at the formal inquiry, and a good administrator will help you decide if this is the right residence for your parent. As you speak with the administrator, do you get the impression she will be available following your parent's admission when you have questions or concerns? Does she seem genuinely interested in your parent? Are you being asked the right questions? Does she have time to listen to your story? Or does she just keep repeating, "Don't worry, we can take care of that"?

Were you able to meet the director of nurses? As overseer of your parent's medical plan of care, she will have the most knowledge about your parent's daily medical requirements. If they say she's busy, ask to say hello for a minute. If she's not approachable now, will she be approachable when you need her?

Trust is a two-way street. As an administrator, I believe it is important for a family to feel comfortable with me. It is equally important that I feel comfortable with the family. In many cases, the admission of a parent to a nursing home is the beginning of a relationship that will last many years. Together, you and the facility staff will walk your parent through his final years, through quiet days as well as troublesome days. Taking the time to do a thorough inquiry will ensure this process takes place in a peaceful, supportive manner.

16 ❧ MORE THINGS YOU SHOULD KNOW ABOUT BEFORE ADMITTING

"I wish I'd brought a tape recorder," sighed Tony. "Since I turned seventy-eight, my memory isn't what it used to be. I had no idea there was so much to learn before I move my mother into a nursing home."

Relocation of any kind takes planning, time, and perseverance. The following are additional points of information needed prior to the actual move-in date. Understanding the challenge of the new environment will help ease the process.

1. The Best Time to Admit
2. The Attending Physician
3. The Podiatrist
4. Dental Care
5. The Use of Restraints
6. The Diaper Policy
7. Catheter Use
8. Visiting Hours

1. The Best Times to Admit: *Not* at Night, *Not* on a Weekend

"I've never lived through anything like it," began an exasperated Ryan. His uncle Stephen had been released from the hospital to a nursing home after being diagnosed with a brain tumor. "I waited at that hospital for *twelve hours* on Friday! The doctor didn't write the discharge order until three in the afternoon. Then, a nurse explained that we'd still have to wait for the ambulance because the company was backlogged. What time do you think we finally arrived?" Before I could answer, he exclaimed, "*Ten-thirty at night!* By then, uncle Stephen was in pain, but they couldn't give him any medication without contacting the nursing home doctor assigned to him. The new guy didn't return the nursing home's call until Saturday morning. To make matters worse, my uncle needed a special air mattress for delicate skin, and no one could deliver one until Monday. There was no one in administration to help us figure out these problems. Poor uncle Stephen has suffered needlessly for three days. Stella, help me get him out of there!"

Every new arrival at a nursing home should be made to feel welcome, special, and secure. However, there seems to be a complete disregard for timing and for the comfort of the patient when a hospital discharges to a long-term care facility. *No nursing home is equipped to carry out a proper admission after six P.M.* It is unlikely an administrator will be there to help you through the process. The director of nurses will not be present to assess your parent's medical and emotional needs. On admission, the attending physician is required to verify the patient's medical orders, but after six in the evening, he will have to be paged. Until he has verified the prescription orders, the pharmacy will be unable to deliver the medications.

There is an art to the admission process. After thirty-seven years of nursing home experience, I can testify that admitting a resident at night, on weekends, or on holidays is a setup for disaster, and I actively discourage it. My policy frequently flies in the face of discharge planners at local hospitals, *but the primary concern should be the welfare and comfort of the residents.*

If questions arise during the relocation process—and they will—the people best qualified to answer them are usually available Monday through Friday. Of course, a nursing home should run smoothly on Saturdays and Sundays, but the admission process is special, and it requires the expertise of the administrator and the director of nurses. When they are involved, they can defuse the anxiety and worries of the family, making the admission smoother and easier for everyone. Even a Friday-morning admission does not give the resident and the family time to become oriented to what is initially a foreign environment. Nor does it give the nursing staff time to create and implement an individualized plan of care, which is critical for the comfort and security of the resident.

If the resident is being admitted from home or from assisted living, your best chance for a successful admission will be late morning or early afternoon between Monday and Thursday. This is because the day shift has the flexibility to focus on welcoming a new resident and family. Inquire about the facility's admission protocol. If a welcoming staff member is not part of their admission process, ask if someone can come out to the car or ambulance and welcome your parent. If you arrive around three in the afternoon, bear in mind this is the time when the staff is sharing pertinent information from one shift to the next and they are not available to be actively involved in an admission for about half an hour. During the three to eleven P.M. shift, the "welcomers" will no longer be on duty. The smaller staff will be stretched to give your parent the attention she deserves.

Once your parent's plan of care is in place, there is still a learning curve for the resident, the family, and the staff. The first few hours and days are the most critical. When is the best time to admit? Not at night. Not on a weekend. Preferably, not even at shift change.

2. The Attending Physician

For nursing homes, individual states require that the attending physician see the resident within a certain number of days following admission. In California, for example, the resident must be seen within seventy-two hours and then monthly thereafter. The facility itself will receive a "deficiency" from government inspectors if the physician does not visit in a timely manner. Ask your parent's attending physician if he can commit to visiting your parent every month in the nursing home. In my experience, the majority of attending physicians are unable to make the commitment. If your parent's doctor cannot do so, ask the facility if they have someone to recommend. Be sure to ask the following questions about the new doctor:

- Does the physician return calls the same day? The administrator or the director of nurses will know. Will the physician speak with the family when decisions need to be made? (Choose *one* family member to act as spokesperson; it is easier on both the physician and the family.)

- How comfortable is the new physician following the directives set forth in your parent's durable power of attorney for health care? Make sure he is supportive of palliative and hospice care, if that is your parent's choice.

3. The Podiatrist

With age, toenails become thick, striated, and brittle, which makes trimming a challenge. Skin surrounding the nail bed is easily bruised or nicked. Because most of the elderly are prone to poor blood circulation, these injuries to the feet can take a long time to heal. For diabetics, even a small sore can become painful and lead to infection.

Every facility has a contract with a podiatrist, and an appointment with your parent is covered by Medicare every sixty days. Be sure your parent is on the list to be assessed by this physician. HMO recipients can only be seen by the HMO-approved podiatrist, who is unlikely to make nursing home visits. Because of this, HMO families frequently choose to pay privately for the facility's podiatrist.

4. Dental Care

Every nursing home has a contract with a local dentist for routine and emergency care. Again, be sure your parent is on the list for an evaluation shortly after admission and approximately every six months thereafter. Dental care is not a Medicare-covered service.

5. The Use of Restraints

The use of restraints, whether physical or chemical, is an emotionally charged subject with families as well as with health-care providers. Since each facility will have its own philosophy, ask for a clear explanation.

Physical Restraints. It is not uncommon for families to say, "We'll take the risk of Mom falling—there's no way we want her restrained." To restrain or not should be the family's decision. Facilities are not allowed to arbitrarily restrain a resident for staff convenience. Before use of a restraint is implemented, an interdisciplinary team must assess safety issues. For example, they may find your parent to be at high risk for falls due to unsteady gait, impaired vision, or diminished judgment. If they recommend a safety belt or "lap buddy," a doctor's order is required as well as the permission of the resident or family. The family will be asked to sign a form acknowledging that they are aware of the recommendation and that they accept or decline the decision. If they decline, the use of a restraint cannot be ordered. If you feel a restraint is no longer necessary, ask the staff to reassess its use.

Chemical Restraints. Much has been written about the overuse of antianxiety medications, antidepressants, tranquilizers, and psychotropic medications. Admonitions not to "drug your parent," and warnings that "drugs will change your parent's personality" frequently prevent families from considering the benefits of chemical intervention. Nonetheless, if your parent exhibits agitated behavior or physical outbursts, her life is far from peaceful. It can be inhumane not to use chemical restraints if in fact they can reduce the anger, fear, depression, paranoia, or agitation that a resident is experiencing.

Since dosage and duration of use differs from person to person, standard medical practice is to "start slow and start low." An evaluation by a geriatric psychiatrist or a physician experienced in caring for the elderly should precede the use of any chemical restraint.

Alan, Dan, and Gina. "I don't have a problem using psychotropic medication for Dad," explained Dan, about his eighty-nine-year-old father, Alan. "Dad believed my mother was having an affair with the local pharmacist. Every time she went to the drugstore, Dad became angry. When his doctor recommended an antianxiety medication, my sister Gina flatly refused to consider 'mind-altering medications,' as she refers to them. She insisted, 'He's not crazy, Danny. He just gets a little mixed up sometimes.' But Dad's fantasy got worse. Even though Mom was standing right there in the room, he would lament that she was in New York with the pharmacist for the weekend. He didn't recognize her and refused to believe anything we said. Dad was miserable, and all my sister could say was, 'Try to reason with him. This will pass.'

"One morning at five A.M., Mom called me in tears," Dan continued. 'Your father is convinced there are roaches coming out of the bathtub, and he's trying to kill them with bug spray. Danny, there are no roaches and I can't get him back in bed!'

"The next day, I accompanied Mom and Dad to a geriatric psychiatrist recommended by his doctor. The psychiatrist ordered lab tests and an MRI and started Dad on a small dose of an antidepressant along with an antianxiety medication. 'Your sister will not be happy,' Mom murmured as we drove home.

"When the doctor asked us how Dad was doing a week later, Mom replied that the imaginary bugs were still frightening him. The doctor increased the medication. During the next week," Dan went on, "Dad's behavior began to improve. Even Gina admitted that life was more peaceful. The bugs disappeared, and Dad's episodes of unpredictable anger decreased."

"I really gave Dan a hard time," Gina later confessed. "Psychotropic drugs are such a hot-button subject. I should have listened more and given directions less. These medications have been a lifesaver for all of us."

6. The Diaper Policy

Approximately 60 percent of residents in long-term-care facilities are incontinent of urine. Each resident should be checked every two hours by the nursing staff, and changed as needed. This schedule should be in effect twenty-four hours a day.

Disposable diapers are available that supposedly need to be changed only every twelve hours; however, the discomfort level, loss of dignity, and risk of infection make these diapers unacceptable. Review with the administrator the diaper system used in the facility.

7. Catheters Use

A catheter is a sterile tube that is inserted through the urethra into the bladder and which drains urine into a plastic container. This device should be used only for specific physiological problems such as enlarged prostate, cancer of the bladder, or urinary retention. Catheters can be a great benefit when necessary but are high risk for infection. In addition, they can be uncomfortable, become clogged, and cause pain. Should your parent be admitted from the hospital with a catheter, ask the director of nurses if it is still necessary and how soon it can be removed. A catheter should never be used merely because the resident is incontinent, bedridden, or confined to a wheelchair.

8. Visiting Hours

Every facility posts visiting hours—typically ten A.M. to seven P.M. If your family has special needs, how flexible are the hours? Even though Bernadette has a difficult commute to downtown Los Angeles, she runs in every morning at seven for a quick visit to see her one-hundred-year-old mother. She says, "I know she doesn't know

I'm here, but I know I'm here." Can the facility you are considering accommodate you? If your parent is critically ill, you should be allowed to visit twenty-four hours a day.

9. The Beauty Shop System

If the facility has a beauty shop on the premises, you will find it is a very busy place. The beautician and manicurist may be employees of the facility or independent contractors. Ask the administrator if they are paid at the time of the visit, or if the charge is added to the monthly bill. How is tipping handled? Are standing appointments recommended, or should you schedule as needed? Will staff members see that your parent arrives on time? Asking these questions ahead of time can eliminate misunderstandings in the future.

10. The Resident's Wardrobe

Provide clothing that your parent currently prefers to wear during the day at home. Be mindful that it will be washed in hotter water than you would use at home, so permanent press is best. Clothing that requires dry cleaning is not advisable. Garments with snaps fare better than those with zippers or buttons. In the nursing home, sweats are by far the most comfortable to wear and the easiest to get on and off. Your parent should have at least ten days' worth of clothing.

Will the facility be responsible for marking your parent's name on clothing? Look over the wardrobe from time to time to see if it needs remarking. The laundry pen may say "indelible," but when the name fades after many washes in hot water, items will end up in the wrong closet.

11. The Laundry System

Are you allowed to do your parent's laundry if you choose? How often should you pick it up? Who will provide the hamper? If your parent is incontinent of bowel and bladder, allow the facility to be responsible for all laundry. Soiled clothing placed in a hamper can cause offensive odors to permeate the area. It must be removed from the room as soon as the resident is changed.

In institutional laundries, there will be misplaced clothing and errors in sorting. While small items such as socks and underwear are difficult to keep track of, a cooperative staff will make an effort to hunt down a missing article of clothing by searching the resident's room. (If you discover that laundry is your main concern, you are probably in a good facility!)

12. The Tipping Policy

Some books recommend tipping the staff. I disagree. When families notice a particular nurse's aide who develops a relationship with their parent, it is normal to want to thank this person with a monetary gift. Most likely they believe tipping guarantees that the nurse's aide will keep a closer eye on their parent. However, an attitude may develop on the part of those who are not given a tip and feelings may be hurt, which was certainly not your intention. Families tend to tip only the staff they see. Many of the people who care for your parent are behind the scenes: the late-night shift, the dietary staff, housekeepers, and maintenance personnel.

I am frequently asked how to show appreciation to the staff. Several years ago, we established an Employee Christmas Fund. Donations are collected from the families and then divided equally among the entire staff. If you want to express thanks during the year, cookies, popcorn, or pizza for each shift will always be enjoyed.

If there is a no-tipping policy, respect it. Think before you put a staff member in an awkward position. Our staff knows accepting a tip is grounds for dismissal.

13. Leaving Cash with Your Parent

For many residents, having their own money represents freedom and independence. They may leave money on the table not because they need it, but because they like to know it is there.

Suzanne gave her mother $50 which soon turned up missing. By the time we found it in the tip of her mother's shoe, relationships of trust had been sorely tested. Suzanne temporarily lost faith in the staff, and the staff felt uncomfortable even though no accusations had been made. When I asked Suzanne why she had given her mother so much cash, she replied, "Mom begged me for it. I know I should have used common sense."

If your parent has experienced memory loss, do not leave money in her room. Petty cash can be placed in the administration office and used as needed. This prevents putting staff in a position where they may be tempted or unjustly suspected. I encourage residents to keep no more than $10. Even then, keep in mind, it may be misplaced.

14. Ordering Medications

If you understand the facility policy on ordering prescriptions before your parent arrives, it will be one less thing to worry about on admission day. Letting the facility order the medications will be easier. In accordance with state laws, you have the right to continue to use your current pharmacy to supply your parent's prescriptions, but you will be responsible to meet your state's pharmaceutical regulations. The rules can be confusing. For example, in California, any medication we receive must be labeled with the specific patient's name, the doctor's name, the number of pills dispensed, the name and strength of the medication, the expiration date, and exact directions. Since state laws vary, ask the facility you choose to explain the regulations.

If you decide to supply prescriptions yourself, find out who is responsible for ordering and reordering medications at the facility. *On a weekly basis*, ask this person, "Does Dad need any of his prescriptions refilled?" Planning ahead to refill prescriptions on time is essential. I recommend having at least a five-day supply on hand in case of emergency. By federal law, each medicine ordered for your parent must be in the facility's medication cart at all times. If you use a mail-order pharmacy, it can take ten days for delivery. Families get busy. They order the medications but forget to pick them up. Or they go on vacation. Since it is not uncommon for residents to require ten to fifteen different medications, keeping the facility stocked with each one can prove overwhelming to the individual family member.

In some states, emergency medications, such as antibiotics or drugs used to treat severe pain, nausea, diarrhea, and agitation, must be available within one hour of the time ordered. This is a difficult rule for most people to comply with. Families who supply routine medications themselves often direct the facility to take care of emergency requirements.

If you supply over-the-counter medications, you must deliver them in unopened, original containers. Products such as Milk of Magnesia, Tylenol, multivitamins, calcium, or Fleet's enemas are more costly if the nursing home orders them for you because there is a delivery charge from the pharmacy. You can purchase them less expensively at bulk-price stores. However, state and federal regulations for nursing homes are again exceptionally strict. If the doctor orders Tylenol for pain, and you bring in Extra-Strength Tylenol, the facility can only accept it if they call the doctor and receive a new order specifying "extra-strength." If the doctor prescribes a multivitamin, and you bring in a multivitamin with minerals, again, a new order is required. These rules are frustrating for everybody, so familiarize yourself with them to eliminate surprises.

15. Hearing Aids and Dentures: Now You See 'Em... Now You Don't

Placed and removed 365 days a year, hearing aids and dentures seem to have a life of their own. Frequently the front office gets a call from the kitchen, saying, "There's a denture on a tray. Who's missing one?" Hearing aids fall on the floor and get crushed. Dentures are placed in a Kleenex box "for safekeeping," only to have the box thrown away. One resident parked her hearing aid in the toe of her shoe. We have found these items in the trash can, in candy boxes, floating in the toilet, and in neighboring residents' pockets.

If your parent is unable to remove a hearing aid and place it in the case, trust me, it will get lost. Left in during sleep, it may fall into the bedding, get bundled up, and sent out with the laundry. Often, residents take out their hearing aids because they pick up background noise, such as several people talking at once. If your parent has dementia and removes her hearing aid, we recommend you return it to the nurses' station when your visit is over. I am aware that the initial response to this plan is, "But my mother should be able to hear all the time!" I agree. However, hearing aids are expensive and caregiving requires flexibility. Keeping hearing aids and batteries at the nurses' station means they will be available when needed. Some families have successfully used an Amplified Listener, a little black box that hangs around the neck. Worn with earphones, it amplifies sound and functions as a hearing aid. It is available from Radio Shack.

Lost dentures are so common in nursing homes that you should ask the dentist to have your parent's name engraved on them. For some residents with dementia, it may not be realistic to wear them all day long.

Missing hearing aids and dentures are a frequent cause of misunderstanding between families and care facilities. Talk to the staff and come up with a workable solution.

16. Developing a Cooperative Game Plan

Since caregiving facilities are most successful when families and staff work as a team, devise a game plan for special needs. If your mother is unable to turn on the TV to watch *Wheel of Fortune,* designate a family member to call the nurses' station every night and remind them to turn it on for her. In time, you will discover that the staff is anticipating your call and has already turned on the TV. One woman asked that her father fall asleep every night listening to his favorite classical radio station. A clock radio was our solution.

Because of staff rotation, employees' days off, and new nurse's aides, some requests are difficult to handle on a daily basis. Misunderstandings happen easily and can lead to tension between family and staff. In extreme cases, I have seen staff avoid certain family members whose demands were unrealistic. A goal of good communication is understanding what is practical; the *art* of good communication is negotiation and flexibility. Be sure to address requests or complaints to the right person. Do not take a problem to a nurse's aide or a housekeeper. Check with administration so that they can direct you to the best person to handle your request.

Good Questions Lead to Good Decisions. Finding the right facility for your parent is not always easy. As you visit facilities, use the inquiry process (see Chapter 15) to ask pointed questions, and evaluate the manner in which they are answered. The education you receive, added to your own intuitive sense of how the facility feels to you, will prepare you to make a decision with a sense of control and confidence.

You cannot plan for every eventuality when admitting your parent to a nursing home or an assisted-living facility. There will always be unexpected details and decisions. How the staff responds to your concerns with workable solutions sets the tone for a successful family/staff partnership. Meanwhile, the more you know and plan ahead, the more comfortable you will be making the transition.

17 ❧ CPR: THE MOST MISUNDERSTOOD CONCEPT IN LONG-TERM CARE

"**S**tella," Dr. Hamilton barked at me as he filled out admission papers for his ninety-two-year-old mother, "I don't understand why you're asking me whether I want CPR for my mother. If she gets sick, I want everything done for her. You should know that."

As we sat at my desk laboring through the required forms, Dr. Hamilton's irritation was obvious. During the past twenty years, he had admitted numerous residents to our nursing home. But today he was simply a son dealing with the powerful emotions that surface on the day of admission.

Because CPR (cardiopulmonary resuscitation) is one if the most misunderstood subjects that I discuss with families, I did not look forward to reviewing it with a physician, especially Dr. Hamilton. I could see that he, like many health-care professionals, was failing to grasp the implications of CPR in regard to the elderly.

"If Mom needs oxygen, of course I want her to have it," he continued, still sounding agitated.

"Has your mother signed a power of attorney for health care form?" I gently inquired.

"Yes, and I'm her designated agent," he answered. "We want no heroics or aggressive measures," he quickly added.

"If your mother's heart stops," I asked gently, "do you want us to attempt to restart it?"

"Stella, if her heart stopped, it would mean she had died. Why would I want you to restart it?"

"That is why I asked about CPR," I cautiously continued. "CPR is an emergency method that can only be used if a person's heart or breathing has stopped. Only then would we begin resuscitation."

Dr. Hamilton sat looking down at the form in front of him. Then he wrote, "No CPR" in bold letters, underlining it three times.

"I should have let you finish explaining the form to me," he added quietly. "I wasn't thinking. No, Stella, I do not want CPR if my mother's heart stops."

As I reminded Dr. Hamilton, CPR only comes into play once the heart has stopped and the patient has died. The overall health of the patient is a major factor in determining the appropriateness of the procedure. Another factor is how long the heart has been stopped. For example, if you saw your friend collapse on the golf course and his heart stopped beating, you would naturally begin CPR—he was healthy enough to be on the golf course and resuscitation efforts could begin immediately. However, such situations rarely exist in long-term care. Residents are likely to be infirm or elderly, and they are often discovered in bed, without vital signs. If more than four minutes have elapsed since the patient's heart stopped beating, brain damage will have occurred.

CPR: What Really Happens

Once CPR is initiated, it takes on a life of its own. If your parent is discovered without a heartbeat, the staff will place her on the floor or slip a cardiac board beneath her because they need a hard surface. Then, one nurse will begin external heart massage, a vigorous and forceful pumping action. At the same time, another nurse will begin mouth-to-mouth breathing. The force of the procedure often causes severe bruising and fractured ribs, which in some cases may puncture the lungs and damage the liver.

As soon as the nurses begin CPR, the staff is required to call 911. Paramedics will transport your mother in an ambulance to the emergency room, where everything possible will be done to resuscitate her. Unless you have previously requested "No CPR," it becomes the responsibility of the nursing home, the paramedics, and the hospital to keep your mother alive.

The emergency room may try to defibrillate her with electric shock paddles. She will probably be connected to a ventilator to help her breathe. After the emergency room has stabilized her, she will be transferred to intensive care, where she will be hooked up to an IV with multiple medications.

Many who survive these circumstances die within a few hours or days. For elderly or seriously ill patients, actual survival to a hospital discharge is less than 5 percent.

Families frequently ask me: "What if Mom needs oxygen? What if she's choking? I don't want her to suffer." Please bear in mind, if your mother's heart is beating, she will receive oxygen and any medications needed for comfort, and her doctor will be notified.

CPR DOCUMENTATION

Orders for "No CPR" relate *only* to CPR, not to other treatments such as those for pain or shortness of breath. Other names for orders restricting resuscitation are "DNR" (do not resuscitate) and "no code" (used in hospitals). In a nursing home, CPR forms must be discussed with families at the time of admission. If the resident or family decides against resuscitation, the family signs a form stating "No CPR." The doctor then co-signs the form and writes an order on the resident's chart.

In assisted living also, DNR forms should be discussed during the admission process. An advance directive is not enough for paramedics. After your parent (or family member) and the doctor sign the form, it becomes part of your parent's file. Should you notice your parent declining in health while in assisted living, it would be helpful to discuss with the administrator putting the DNR form on the wall by your parent's door, with the words "For Paramedics." This gives notice and legal authority to staff and paramedics not to perform CPR. In the absence of this form, medical personnel will always proceed with resuscitation.

Laws governing the content of DNR documents vary from state to state. You can obtain official preprinted forms through the state or county medical association, the bar association, or a local Area Agency on Aging.

Health-Care Professionals Have a Responsibility

Admissions personnel are required to ask, "Do you want CPR for your parent?" This question is unintentionally misleading; it prompts a belief that CPR may offer a real benefit. Thus, the family may feel obligated to request CPR. On the other hand, signing a Do Not

Resuscitate form can leave a family feeling guilty and neglectful. As one daughter told me, "I feel like I'm saying, 'Sure, go ahead and let my mother die.'"

CPR is an intense, undignified treatment with a high probability of extended suffering. I believe the admitting facility has a professional responsibility to review and explain the exact implications of CPR. When your parent's wishes are known, having a DNR in place means that no critical decision awaits you when you may be emotionally unprepared; it means that you have accepted that your parent may die a natural death and that you do not wish to prolong her life artificially, but rather to allow a dignified, end-of-life experience.

18 ✐ THE FIRST TWENTY-FOUR HOURS

The day of admission to a nursing home can be highly emotional for both you and your parent. Even though the decision has been made, the following doubts may still be racing through your mind:

> *"Why do we have to make this move?"*
> *"Am I really doing the right thing?"*
> *"How can I leave her here?"*
> *"What if she refuses to stay?"*
> *"Will she forgive me?"*
> *"What if she hates the food?"*
> *"Will the staff understand how to take care of her?"*

You may also find yourself experiencing the most difficult-to-understand feeling of all—relief. ("Thank heaven I'm not totally responsible for Mom anymore. I'll finally have some time for myself.") When caregivers experience relief from the day-to-day care of their parents, they often feel guilty precisely *because* they feel relieved.

This jumble of emotions is a normal part of relocating your parent. Oddly, talking about your sense of guilt is socially acceptable, but expressing your relief is not. We seem to feel that in order for the move to be the right decision, it has to benefit only your parent; if it benefits us as well, perhaps there was a selfish motive. Find someone you trust, preferably someone who has gone through the same experience, and confide your feelings. You may continue to feel guilty that you could not give your mother the care she needed, but as you accept that the decision truly was in her best interest, guilt over the relief you feel will dissipate.

Angie and Her Mother

"Am I selfish for wanting to reclaim my life?" asked Angie as we drank coffee in my office. "I've been dreading this day. In a practical sense, I know moving Mom was necessary—I couldn't give her the care she needed anymore—but leaving her now scares me. She's aware enough to realize she's not at home. I was just beginning to feel in control of the situation. Now, all my guilt and doubts are coming back."

"The admission appeared to go smoothly," I commented.

"It did," she nodded tentatively. "I followed your recommendations. Yesterday, I came in to fill out the admission forms ahead of time. While I was here, I put up Mom's favorite pictures and spread her afghan on the bed. Today, just as you predicted, Precious and Kimo, your two little house dogs, came running out to meet Mom as she was getting out of the car. That broke the tension; she loves dogs. I hated to leave her so soon, but I have to get to work."

I came around the desk to sit beside Angie. "Did you say goodbye to your mother before you left?"

"No," Angie sighed, "I just slipped out of the room and didn't go back. I didn't want to make things worse, and she'd probably forget I said good-bye anyway." Catching my glance, Angie threw her hands in the air and exclaimed, "Okay...you want me to go back and say good-bye, right? Stella, I just don't want to make her sad."

"Angie," I smiled. "All the things you've just shared with me are normal, natural reactions. Wanting to reclaim your life is not selfish. Have a little compassion for yourself, and understand that you, too, are going through a big change."

"I didn't think of it that way," she said thoughtfully.

"The first day is seldom without difficult moments. Don't be distressed if your mother expresses sadness or even anger during this transition. If you allow your mother to vent her emotions, it will help her. Some residents take a while to adjust."

"I'm glad we arrived before lunch," Angie commented. "Being introduced to the ladies at her dining table made her feel included."

"The real key to adjustment is time. Did you sit down with the director of nurses and go over the kind of care you've been providing for your mom?"

Angie nodded. "She asked me millions of questions—who gave the care, how it was provided, what worked, and what didn't. She asked about any problems Mom might have, like allergies or sleeping difficulties."

"It's a great opportunity to share with the nursing staff as much information as you can," I reminded her. "We want to know your mom as a person, not merely as a room number. The more we know, the faster we can make her comfortable with us."

Angie frowned. "I'm still feeling panicky about whether I made the right decision."

"That's why planning for today was so important," I reminded her. "It's hard to think clearly when you're feeling fearful or guilty. Your mom needs twenty-four-hour care, which you are physically unable to continue. Try to accept your limitations without judging yourself too harshly."

"Easier said than done," she replied.

"Angie," I continued, "by providing a professional staff to care for her, you have made a truly responsible choice. You will remain a caregiver for your mom, and you will continue to play an active role in her care. Through regular visits, you will be her advocate. I cannot stress enough the importance of your role in the success of your mom's adjustment."

"I'm ready," Angie said as she stood up. "I'll go give Mom a kiss and say good-bye."

"It's not easy, Angie," I said, "but let her know you care, and that you'll be back tomorrow. We'll remind her if she asks for you."

How Long Should I Stay?

There are experts who recommend staying as long as you can on the first day. Others say, "Leave at the earliest opportunity and don't come back for a few days." Blanket statements will not work for everyone. If it feels right, you should plan on staying for an hour or two, and then leave. However, because of family dynamics, a parent's feelings, and your own insecurities, each admission is a unique experience. I have advised some families to leave before lunch, others to stay two or three hours. I have even requested that some leave and come back an hour or two later. How long you should stay the first day will depend on your needs and those of your parent.

Give the Staff a Chance

Keep in mind that when your family is present, the staff will usually stay out of the room to give you privacy. If your family visits for five hours on the first day, the staff will not immediately bond with your parent. This may not seem like a problem—why couldn't they get to know your parent the following day? But if your parent hasn't connected with the staff, and everybody leaves at once, who will fill that first immediate void?

Allow the staff to establish your parent's new schedule as soon as possible. This is vitally important for the resident with dementia, who will respond well to routine. If your parent gets involved in the very first activity following admission, that routine will have begun. As a result, your parent may not be as anxious when you leave. Families who spend many hours visiting on the first day may be unconsciously telegraphing their own uncertainty about the relocation.

Don't be frightened if your "perfect" admission results in tears or anxiety on the part of your parent. Questions such as "What am I doing here?" "How did I get here?" "How long am I staying?" can be a normal part of the process. Some people take two days to adjust. Others may take two weeks or two months.

Saying Good-bye the First Day

On the first day, let the staff know when you are leaving, so they can monitor how your parent is doing. Like Angie, families frequently ask me if they should "just disappear." No. Always take formal leave of your parent, whether they will remember it or not. If your parent is alert, it is especially important for her to understand when you will return. When your family visits as a group, leave in shifts to avoid a sudden silence after all the talk and activity.

The First Night

By the time you are ready to leave on admission day, you should feel less anxious than when you arrived. If you are still uneasy, touch base with the administrator or the director of nurses. They will be able to explain how they will help your parent settle in for the evening. It is common to experience anxiety the first night. If you do, call the charge nurse to see how your parent is adjusting. Sometimes, talking with your parent on the phone will make both of you feel more secure and connected. For others, it can start the process of asking to go home all over again. The charge nurse can assess how your parent is doing and advise you.

Quality care depends on staff and family members communicating and working together throughout the adjustment time. It starts on the first day.

"My sister who lives out of state says I should visit Mom every day," Darcy lamented, "but I'm the only one who took care of her for six long years. The stress is jeopardizing my marriage. Now my husband says I need to cut back for my own health. My sister may say I'm letting our mother down, but half the time Mom won't know I've been here anyway. So who is the visit really for?"

Families frequently ask how often they should visit. It is important to go with your intuition and feel comfortable with your decision. In Darcy's case, I suggested she start by visiting three times a week. As long as she felt comfortable being away for a couple of days, it would help her mother and the staff get to know one another. Dementia residents feel safe within a highly structured environment. The sooner they adjust to a routine, the sooner feelings of comfort and security can take root. Darcy did take a few well-deserved days off, and to her relief, her mother never realized she had been gone.

An alert resident, on the other hand, may benefit from frequent visits during the first weeks. Cheryl sat in my office on the day of her mother's admission. "My sister Becky and I spent the night at Mom's house," she told me. "We thought it would help stabilize the emotions we were all feeling. This morning we all laughed and cried as we got ready. In Mom's new room, Becky arranged the clothes and toiletries, while I worked with the movers who were delivering the bedroom furniture. By the time the room had been personalized with her things, Mom had joined a group of ladies for lunch. Everything went along pleasantly, but as we prepared to leave, Mom pleaded, 'Girls, don't leave. I'm not ready to say good-bye.'"

During the first days following admission, the alert resident will need the security of knowing that she has not been deserted and that you will continue to be actively involved in her life. The routine established by the facility will be enhanced by the structure you give with your calls and visits.

The More You Visit, the Easier It Gets

Quality nursing homes *always* welcome visitors. Initially, family members may be intimidated by the new environment. Adult children of dementia patients may fear the disappointment of not being recognized by their parent. Seeing your mom out of her usual setting can be disorienting. Suddenly, she looks older, more frail. Lost in a sea of white-haired ladies, she looks like one of "them" and not like "Mom."

"How can I relate to her now?" a woman once asked me. The answer: Visit regularly. The more you visit, the more comfortable you will be with your parent, the facility, and the staff members.

Be prepared to experience different kinds of visits. There will be happy, meaningful visits, along with sad, possibly disturbing ones, but each visit will help continue the family bond and reassure your parent that he is loved. If at times you truly have no desire to visit, go with your feelings. Visiting out of a sense of duty will only make you feel pressured and guilty. When you are under stress, your parent is likely to sense it. Wait until you are in the right frame of mind.

Visiting is a commitment. Give a date and time only if you feel able to keep the appointment. Alert residents look forward to visits, so if you must cancel, call at the earliest convenience. What is common courtesy becomes imperative when a nursing home resident is looking forward to company.

Respect Your Parent's New Routine

Because of different work and home responsibilities, available visiting time will vary from family to family. However, it is necessary to remember that your parent will also have routines and schedules that are an important part of his day; for example, an exercise class involves socialization with other residents. If you can visit when your parent is in his room between activities and meals, the quiet, personal visit will truly add to his day. Obtain a copy of the activity schedule and consult with staff members about the best hours to visit.

Check in with the Staff

Upon entering the facility, let the staff at the nurses' station know who you are and whom you are visiting. Ask if there are any changes you should know about. If you know in advance that your father was participating in activities all day or that he worked with a physical therapist, for example, you won't be alarmed if he seems tired.

The more the staff gets to know you, the better it is for your parent. If you treat your parent and the staff with respect and thoughtfulness, your parent will become highly visible on the staff radar. Research confirms that residents who have more visitors have a more positive nursing home experience than those who have fewer visitors.

Schedule Different Times for Large Families

If you have a large family, schedule visits at different times of the day or week. Even two visitors at a time can be overwhelming to those who are hard of hearing or have dementia. Too often, family members do not speak directly to the parent but rather chat among themselves. Come to spend time talking with your parent, not to visit the rest of your family. Such gatherings frequently result in everyone having a good time except the parent.

Lower Your Voice

Many visitors think that the louder they talk, the better the elderly resident will hear. In fact, dropping your voice to a lower tone and speaking slowly is far more effective. Choose a quiet area to visit, moving away from background noise.

Brief Visits Can Be Successful

If your parent is alert, she may try to be a good host by keeping a conversation meaningful and interesting, but this can be tiring. Keeping your visit short—ten to twenty minutes—will take the pressure off both of you. If your parent has dementia, just a few minutes of holding her hand will let her know she is accepted and loved.

Photo Albums Are Almost Always a Hit

The photo album reminds the alert parent of her ongoing connection to the family. For the cognitively impaired resident, who is likely to be more comfortable in the past, the album is a pleasant reminder of past relationships and occasions. Large, clear family photographs are best. Some families bring in videotapes or DVDs of grandchildren talking and singing.

Children Are Always Welcome

Bringing children to a facility is a win/win situation since all residents and staff benefit from the smiles and laughter of little ones. Your parent can play simple games like cards or dice with your children without worrying about following the rules. Families can also bring in drawings and pictures of grandchildren to place on the walls and closet doors to brighten up their parents' rooms. It is beneficial to let your children see that a close relationship with Grandma is important. My mother once remarked as my son and I were concluding a visit, "The way you take care of me is a wonderful lesson for Christopher." Take the time to demonstrate that, just like everyone, the elderly need attention and affection.

Treats Are Wonderful

Special foods such as chocolate croissants or perhaps lox and bagels will be a welcome change from your parent's usual diet. Make it something that has always been her favorite. If your parent is on dietary restrictions, request that the registered dietician or doctor assess the diet to allow a treat as often as possible.

When you bring candies, cookies, or fruit, place them in an airtight container because sweets can attract insects. Even quality facilities must work diligently to keep rooms free of ants and other undesirable visitors. For residents who are cognitively impaired, leave treats with the charge nurse or the administration office to be distributed at intervals; otherwise, the treats may be eaten all in one sitting or forgotten altogether.

Make Sure a Car Trip Will Be Worthwhile

If you plan an outing, be sure your parent feels up to it or you may discover early in the trip he is already too exhausted to enjoy himself. Avoid crowded places that can overstimulate your parent. If he is unable to leave the facility, wheel him around the grounds. This activity not only stimulates conversation, it also provides you with an opportunity to observe the care of other patients and get to know the staff better.

Sing!

Walking along the corridor, I often heard singing coming from Room 103. Sarah had been visiting her ninety-four-year-old mother at the nursing home for three years. An only child who never married, Sarah was very devoted to her mother. At first, Sarah had visited once or twice a day, but over the years as the dementia progressed, she had changed her routine to twice a week. "Who thought this is what awaited us?" Sarah shared with me during one of her visits. "Conversation is next to impossible now, but Mom and I have found a different way to communicate—we sit and sing together. While many memories are gone, the songs we love from long ago somehow remain."

According to a study of the effect of music on dementia patients, singing is a valuable source of stimulation—a method of communication that reduces agitation, promotes engagement in activities, and encourages interaction with other people.

"All Dad Does Is Complain"

If your parent targets you with complaints every time you visit, you may feel unappreciated and leave with the impression that your visit accomplished nothing. However, do not withdraw. Sometimes complaining is just a step in the adjustment process during which the resident must feel free to control his environment. It can be a coping technique to verbally express sadness or loneliness. Other causes for nonstop complaining are:

- need for attention
- anger at the loss of independence
- fear of being abandoned by the family
- attempts to control adult children

Even though generally satisfied with a facility and the care their parent is receiving, adult children can find a stream of complaints emotionally overwhelming. Initially, they can be fearful that they have done the wrong thing "abandoning" their parent to "this place." I once asked a resident why she found so much to complain about and what we could do to make things better for her. Without blinking, she answered, "I don't have anything to talk about, so I complain." If your parent complains constantly, always listen. Allow your parent to vent feelings, but set a limit to the complaint time, and then tactfully change the subject. Suggest taking a walk, or ask your parent's advice on a subject about which he is particularly knowledgeable.

To all appearances, Evelyn's admission went smoothly. It was only when her family visited that we found out "nothing was right." The staff observed one type of behavior, the family observed another. At eighty-nine, Evelyn had just left her home of sixty years. During her first week in assisted living, Evelyn ate a balanced diet, attended activities, and took daily walks. She told the staff, "I miss my home, but everyone here is so nice." However, when her daughter Norma came to visit, the food was too salty, the bed too hard, and there was nothing to do. The staff had heard none of these remarks. "Help!" begged Norma.

In such cases, we listen closely to the family and investigate each of their concerns to reassure them that our primary concern is their parent's care and comfort. If your parent says "absolutely everything is wrong" the first few weeks, she is probably still adjusting. If the complaining continues after meaningful attempts have been made to alleviate concerns, it may be an attention-getting device or a fear of being abandoned. It may also be a method of "controlling" adult children and may have nothing whatever to do with the staff or the care being given. Once the underlying cause of complaining is understood, the adult children will have the security of knowing that the complaints and concerns have been addressed.

If you hear a complaint, before you rush to the nurses' station tense and ready for battle, stop and think: Are you dealing with a minor issue or is this a real problem? Are you angry that you had no choice but long-term-care placement? Could you be taking your frustration out on the staff? Consider that you, too, are going through an adjustment process. Think with as clear a head as possible and then communicate the problem to the staff. I am not suggesting that you placate the staff. However, befriending the staff, teaching them who your parent is, and acknowledging their input creates the best scenario. A relationship like this takes time to establish. Remember, they are giving your parent the care that you are no longer able to give. Think of them as part of your team, not as an adversary that must be micromanaged.

Herbert and Margaret. After visiting his eighty-six-year-old mother, Margaret, Herbert dropped by my office. Clearly concerned, he said, "Mom claims your staff pushed her around and tried to drown her yesterday."

When we investigated the problem, the nurse's aide, Naomi, explained that Margaret was incontinent of bowel and bladder and had urgently needed a shower. In second stage dementia, she resisted being changed and bathed. "I did speak to her firmly," said Naomi, "but I had no choice—she needed a bath head to toe." After thirty minutes, Naomi was finally able to coax Margaret into the shower, but the disagreeable episode made Margaret think Naomi was trying to drown her. If Herbert had not explored the complaint, he would have left feeling ineffective, anxious, and probably angry.

When you attempt to decipher exactly what brought about a complaint, consider that your parent's perception of the event may not be entirely accurate (although I have found there is usually an element of fact in each complaint). If the same complaint is frequent and consistent, share this with the director of nurses. She will want to look into it for your benefit and hers. If you feel a legitimate complaint is not being resolved, take your concern to the administrator. Ignoring it will damage your parent's morale and leave you feeling powerless.

Give It Time

Residents adjust to their new environment at their own rate. Our best allies are time and patience. If things aren't going well from your parent's point of view, but you feel comfortable with the staff and the environment, step back, try to be objective, and allow for an adjustment period. (If roommates don't get along, talk to the nursing staff about options.) Some residents slip into the daily routine from the moment they arrive. In my experience, however, the average resident takes about three months to feel secure and satisfied in the new home. If in that time your parent does not feel settled, give it three more months. Meanwhile, work with the staff to eliminate obstacles to your parent's comfort and well-being.

Visiting Your Cognitively Impaired Parent

Visiting a cognitively impaired parent can be sad and frustrating. Remember, *the Alzheimer's patient is always right.* Correcting inaccurate information may anger or embarrass her, and it will certainly exhaust you. Try to listen without reinforcing inaccurate perceptions. As your parent repeats the same story again and again, gently redirect the conversation.

Dee and Fran. The two women had just finished visiting their mothers and were sitting on the patio with me. "It's been a down day for Mom," said Dee. "Just two days ago, we had a lovely visit, but today all she did was ask me the same questions over and over again."

"Dee," I responded, "whether your visit has been meaningful or disheartening, it will have long-term value to you and your mom. The important thing is that you are here for her."

"I wish my mom could speak at all," said Fran, whose mother was in late stage two dementia. "When I visit, I just have a one-sided conversation. I've made peace with myself that I've lost her, but whenever I visit, I feel the loss all over again. I don't know why I visit since she doesn't even know I'm here."

"Visiting your mother is always important," I stressed to both of them. "It reminds everyone on the staff 'this is my mother and she is important to me,' so give yourself credit for being her advocate. Even if the visit feels meaningless to you, the comforting presence of another person is still important to your mother."

Unexpected Relationships Develop

Families who visit frequently develop relationships with other residents and other families. Two daughters of patients in our nursing home became friends and travel companions. A gentleman who visited his aunt met a woman who visited her mother, and a lovely relationship grew that continued long after the death of the two residents. A dentist visiting his father ended up with new clients. This is a natural result of participating in a warm, caring community.

As time goes on, you may find yourself visiting more with the staff or other residents than with your cognitively impaired parent. This is not uncommon. John used to visit his father for ten to fifteen minutes, holding his hand. Then he would come back to the office and visit with the staff, showing them pictures of the grandchildren. After a while, he would go back to see his father for a short while and then say good-bye. John was fulfilling his goal of family involvement with his father and remaining a solid part of the caregiving team.

"Mom Doesn't Want Me to Leave"

At times, concluding a visit may be difficult. Tell your parent up front how long you plan to stay. During your visit, be sure to convey by your words and actions that she is loved, important, and worthwhile. If you plan your departure to coincide with lunch or your mother's visit to the beauty shop, the activity will work as a distraction so that you are not leaving your parent "alone." Because the staff will come to know your parent's preferences, they may be able to give you ideas, such as, "Leave just before the current events class; your mother really enjoys that." If your parent pressures you to stay, acknowledge that parting is difficult for you, too, and remind her what you need to do: "Mom, it's time for me to pick up the kids." Tell her you love her, state when you will be back, and say good-bye.

Share What You've Learned with the Staff

At the end of your visit, check in again with the staff to share any information you may have gathered. Be sure to tell them if you left your parent in an anxious mood or if you observed the beginning symptoms of a cold. The staff sees your parent many times a day, but not for prolonged, one-on-one visits. We have halted many illnesses before they grew worse because of the sharp eyes of our families.

While sharing information with the staff, thank them for their care and concern. Ask their opinion on treats to bring or good times to visit. The staff will feel valued, included, and respected. Finally, have a good attitude about your visit—you want your parent and the staff to be glad you came.

"I'm not staying, Frances! I've changed my mind. Let's go."

"I'm hearing those words in my sleep!" fretted Frances. At eighty-nine, her mother, Janet, suffered from stage two dementia. "She agreed to come," Frances went on, "but I'm afraid that just as all the furniture is moved in, she'll look at me and say, 'Take me home!'"

"If she does, it will not be the time to confront her with agreements she made in the past," I pointed out. "Just because you are right does not mean her fears are not real. Arguing won't change a thing—we need to come up with a plan."

I recommended that Frances and Janet arrive an hour before lunch. If Janet was resistant to her new surroundings, Frances would stay and have lunch with her. "While you wait for lunch," I suggested, "slowly begin to unpack, asking your mother where she would like her belongings. If she says, 'Take me home,' explain again the reasons for the move, without arguing or apologizing. If one reason is to maintain the order and sanity of your own family life, don't be afraid to say so."

I further advised Frances to use the "I" statements technique described in Chapter 4. With "I" statements, you place the burden of the request upon yourself: not "you need to do this," but "I need you to help me with this." On admission day, Frances used this tactic with Janet.

"I need you to help me, Mom," said Frances. "We decided together this was the right move. I am not abandoning you. I worried so much about your being alone in your apartment when I wasn't around. Now you'll have people close by all the time. Let's start by having lunch and learning about your new routine." Before Frances left, she placed a large calendar on the wall and wrote "Frances will be here before lunch" on the next day's date. Because she had a plan, Frances felt in control and did not communicate her own anxiety to her mother.

Owning a home was a hallmark for our parents. Their dream may be to remain in that home. Unfortunately, staying at home beyond the age of safety and security is a prescription for a family crisis. Relocating parents to a well-chosen long-term-care facility may be the best choice.

Freda and Bob. At age seventy-nine, Freda was admitted to a geriatric-psychiatric unit for major depression and Alzheimer's. Her husband, Bob, had been caring for her at home. Their daughter Kay told me, "My father has always been an overbearing man, and now he's angry because Mom's more helpless than ever. Two years ago, she started getting lost in the shopping mall. Once, she walked home, forgetting the car in the parking lot. More and more she was unable to account for how she spent her days, and now she refuses to get dressed or leave the house."

Every time Bob visited Freda at the geriatric-psychiatric unit, she cried and pleaded to go home, leaving both of them frustrated and distressed. At the end of a week, the psychiatric staff recommended that Freda move to an assisted-living facility while Bob continued to live at home.

To avoid a scene between Bob and Freda, Kay arranged for a geriatric care manager to transport her mother from the hospital. Kay had personalized Freda's room with family pictures, a favorite afghan, and a rocking chair. Still, on arrival, Freda announced, "I want to go home." Quickly, the staff stepped in to distract her; they convinced her to attend an exercise-to-music class, which she enjoyed. However, when she returned to her room and saw her pictures, she repeated her desire to go home. Again the staff was able to divert her attention and deal with her anxiety. Once involved in a task, she forgot her concerns. Three days later, Bob visited.

When Freda saw him, she became nearly hysterical, wanting to go home. Angry and defensive, he fumed, "Why did I come? She won't listen to me. She knows I can't take care of her anymore."

Interceding, the activities director invited Freda to help serve coffee. "Come on, Freda, the ladies are waiting for you," she said.

"I'll go," cried Freda, trembling, "but I don't want to."

Bob had seen enough. Turning to me, he stormed, "I'm not coming back—it's too hard to see her like this." Silently, I motioned him over to the patio, where he could observe her unseen as she took part in the activities. Standing outside, he saw that she was pouring coffee and interacting with a group of ladies.

For two months, Bob monitored his wife this way without seeing her face-to-face, watching her from outside the activities room and from a balcony that overlooked her living area. Finally one day he declared, "I'm ready to try again." I recommended that he join her in the afternoon's activities, which he did. The visit went smoothly. As Bob prepared to leave, his eyes were moist.

Smiling at her husband, Freda said, "Now it's your turn to cry.'"

Bob looked at me, shaking his head. "My wife is some lady!" he remarked.

When Your Parent Gets Mean

Cognitively impaired residents can become angry, confused, and frightened during the relocation and adaptation process. What they say to their children can be devastating.

"If you don't take me home, I will never love you again."

"I'm sorry I gave birth to you."

"All you want is my money. I'm calling the police."

"Your father would be so disappointed with how you're treating me."

"Your sister would never have put me here."

Devastating as the remarks are, the parent with dementia is not in control of what he is saying. Remember that you can never win the argument—you can only change the subject or start a new activity to break the train of thought.

Tilly and Barbara. "If you don't take me home, you're no longer my daughter. Don't bother coming back," cried Tilly, a ninety-one-year-old resident, to her daughter Barbara.

"Mom was living in her own apartment," Barbara explained, "but I scheduled the twenty-four-hour care, bought her food, ordered the medications, and paid her bills. In the last ten days, she has fallen four times, and now she's incontinent. Between my job, my husband, and my mother, I can't keep up this pace. Sometimes I feel as old as she is. On top of everything else, she says the meanest things to me."

"Is your mother being mean, Barbara, or is she trying to get your attention so she can gain some control over her life?" I asked. "It is not uncommon for a new resident to have feelings of apprehension, abandonment, and loneliness. As a caregiver, you must understand that her life was pulled out from under her when she left her familiar surroundings."

A few days later, Barbara told me, "I'm a better listener now. I don't try to change her mind; I just let her talk about her anxieties and try to comfort her. Also, I remind her why we made this move and how grateful I am that she was willing to come."

If Barbara had not allowed her mother to vent her feelings, their relationship would have been unpleasantly strained. By listening, Barbara validated her mother's feelings and strengthened their relationship. Further, by her regular visits, she calmed her mother's fear of abandonment.

You May Need to Relocate

Unfortunately, there are facilities that do not deliver quality care. Some situations must be addressed immediately, for example, the use of restraints without your approval, failure to notify you after a fall, mismanagement of medication, or anything else that jeopardizes your parent's safety and quality of life. Take your concerns immediately to the director of nurses or the administrator. If you do not get a satisfactory response, you may need to relocate your parent. Before making such a decision, however, be sure you are being objective and have solid reasons, because a move will be difficult and disruptive for you and for your parent. As exhausting as moving sounds, keep in mind you will be a far more sophisticated consumer than you were on your first foray into long-term care. There is a facility for your parent. Network with friends, health-care professionals, and social workers. You will find the right one.

Geraldine and Martha. "Take me home!" Geraldine, eighty-seven, yelled at her daughter Martha on admission day and on two subsequent visits. Geraldine, diagnosed with Alzheimer's, had her daughter in tears.

"I have to take her home," Martha sobbed. "I can't bear to see her so unhappy."

Martha moved her mother back to her old apartment with the same three caregivers she had employed before. A week later, Martha called me more overwrought than before and described the exchange taking place daily with her mother:

"Take me home!" her mother would yell.

"You are home, Mom," Martha would reassure her.

"My home is 1401 Wyoming," Geraldine would insist. "You know what house I mean."

It turned out 1401 Wyoming had been Geraldine's address as a newlywed sixty-five years earlier. "Home" was a memory of her youth, which no longer existed. Geraldine rejoined us. On occasion, she still asked to go home, but rather than doubting herself, Martha gently responded, "You are home, Mom, and I am here with you." Geraldine's clearest thoughts were of the distant past, and Martha learned to live there with her.

Your own emotional state of mind may cloud a fair appraisal of your parent's care. When you hear "Take me home," listen patiently without arguing, apologizing, or correcting. Allow your parent to vent. Calmly review with your parent (and yourself) the reasons for the move. When appropriate, use distraction methods. Since all residents adjust to their new living arrangements at their own rate, there is no way to predict how quickly your parent will feel at home. Brace yourself for some possible discontent, but realize that if you have done your research, have had an in-depth inquiry with the administrator, and are willing to work with the staff as a team member, you are likely on the road to a successful transition.

After visiting several other nursing homes, Dolores selected our facility for her aunt. "I knew right away this was the place I wanted because of the smiling faces of your staff when I walked in the door. I can feel the high morale."

"Dolores, staff morale is a key indicator of quality care," I confirmed.

"What's your secret?" asked Dolores as she sat down in my office.

"Starting at the bottom," I smiled. "Halfway through nursing school, I was a nurse's aide for three months. I was youthfully idealistic about giving good care. It didn't take long for my enthusiasm to dwindle. I quickly learned that if you were 'just a nurse's aide,' you were at the low end of the totem pole, doing difficult, repetitive, and often unpleasant tasks. I cared for dementia patients, most of whom were unable to thank me. In the afternoon, I left my patients clean, dry, and sitting up;

the next morning, I found them in bed with soiled diapers, mussed hair, and unbrushed teeth. I had to start all over again. Yet for all my hard work, the administrator and the director of nurses never acknowledged my efforts. Nurse's aides were not held in esteem. That experience planted the seeds of my personal philosophy—that the way you treat the people who have hands-on contact with the residents is a reflection of the overall care families can expect for their loved ones. When nurse's aides are treated with respect and appreciation, you can literally see the difference when you walk in the door."

"I never thought much about who was actually taking care of my aunt," Dolores admitted.

"Dolores, it's the CNA—certified nurse's assistant, commonly referred to as a nurse's aide—who has the closest contact with your aunt. The backbone of the nursing home, CNAs are the bottom of the nursing hierarchy. Currently, many CNAs are women who come from economically depressed countries, including Mexico, Central America, India, Korea, and the Philippines. Some work two jobs, and most have families to take care of when they get off work. Unfortunately, since our society doesn't hold the aged in esteem, it naturally follows that we don't respect those who care for them."

One day, a hardworking CNA named Aurora came into my office, crying. "Mrs. Peterson is blaming me for losing her mother's sweater. She is so angry," she wept. "She treats me like a maid. I'm sorry if I said the wrong thing, but I told her, 'I went to school to be a certified nurse's aide—I'm not a maid.' I take care of her mother the best I can, Mrs. Henry, but she always looks down on me with a mean face and complains my English isn't good. I know she'll be in to talk to you about me."

Sitting with Aurora and giving her a chance to calm down, I thanked her for explaining the situation. As she left my office, she turned and said, "Mrs. Peterson is a good daughter to her mother. Just not good to me."

If staff members are treated badly, how can we expect them to treat residents well? Berating Aurora over minor issues will not improve the care she gives to Mrs. Peterson's mother. In more and more states, you will find that English is not the aides' first language. This seems to annoy some families. *I can teach the CNAs English; I cannot teach them respect for the elderly.* An advantage of foreign-born CNAs is that they retain a cultural respect for the elderly, which leads them to treat their patients with gentleness and empathy.

The CNA in a nursing home does not have an easy job. She takes orders from supervisors and endures stress from demanding families while juggling her own personal life. She dresses and undresses her residents, bathes them, and feeds them, often caring for people who have no control over their bowels and bladder. She performs the most intimate tasks of care. It is disheartening to see a CNA with her resident all dressed and ready to go, only to have the resident soil himself, requiring a bath and a total change of clothes. One CNA confided to me, "I go home so tired and I'm sure everyone can smell urine and feces on me. After I shower, I can still smell it." There are times when a resident will try to bite or hit the nurse who changes him. A small task such as brushing teeth can develop into a physical attack. Even the residents' families, feeling helpless over their parents' decline, at times take out their anger and frustration on the aide.

"People think I'm just a worker who cleans up the residents," said Cora. "I work hard. Sometimes I go home with aches and bruises because I have to fight with the residents to care for them. I still need to take care of my children. My husband gets mad at me because all I want to do is sleep. But I am treated with respect here. The charge nurse tells me what to do. The staff developer corrects me. The director of nurses tells me when I've done something wrong. This is part of being a CNA, but they also let me know I've done a good job, and that makes me feel respected and valued for the hard work I do."

The more family members understand who is caring for their parent, the better they will communicate and work as a team. Try to develop a cooperative relationship with the nurses' aide, keeping in mind she may be shy with family members. By being sympathetic regarding the work she does, you may find her more approachable.

Conversely, the CNA must understand the needs and fears of the families, especially at the time of admission. At one of the classes we hold for CNAs, one observant young aide shared with the others, "When they first arrive, the families are worried and scared. Often they don't trust us very much. As the days go by and we get to know each other, they relax and start smiling."

If you think a CNA is not living up to her responsibilities, talk to the director of nurses. Report any behavior that does not meet your expectations. Your input helps everyone.

Death is a constant aspect of nursing home life. Since most residents will live in the nursing home for the rest of their lives, it is likely that a CNA or other staff member will be with them when they die. However long the aide has assisted the resident, she inevitably becomes emotionally involved and experiences grief when the resident dies. But there is not much time for mourning. When the nurse's aide returns the next day, she finds a new resident in the same bed—and the caregiving cycle begins again. All too often, the grief of the nurse is overlooked. As one nurse's aide shared following the death of one of her patients, "Families are sad and distracted when their parent dies. They probably don't know that I'm sad, too, and that I have tried to make it easier for them."

As I looked up, Dolores was almost in tears. "Stella, you're sending a new woman out there. CNAs face real challenges, and I promise I'm not going to add to their daily stress."

Dolores was true to her word. Recognizing the difficult work of the CNAs and giving them respect and recognition for their work, she created a bond instead of a barrier. Considering herself part of the team, she became at ease sharing responsibilities such as feeding her aunt and walking her up and down the hall for exercise. Knowing her aunt was cared for by people she could rely on gave her peace of mind and a sense of community as she and her aunt adjusted to the new environment.

22 ✐ TIME TO THINK ABOUT THE FINAL JOURNEY

"My daughter Annette is so excited that I'm turning ninety-six," laughed Yetta. "She's invited thirty-two family members to our favorite restaurant for lunch. Such a fuss they're making," she said with a smile.

Later that afternoon, I received a call from her daughter. Her voice was troubled, but calm. "Stella," she began, "Mom enjoyed champagne before lunch, followed by her favorite dish, beef Wellington. We all sang 'Happy Birthday,' ate cake, and presented her with a replica of the wedding ring she had lost many years before. The next thing I knew Mom leaned to her left as though she had fainted. We called the paramedics, but she never regained consciousness. She died in the ambulance on the way to the hospital."

What must Yetta have done to earn such a good death—surrounded by family, having just finished her favorite meal? Most of us will not be so lucky.

Marvin and Susie. One day, Marvin and his noticeably pregnant wife, Susie, arrived at my office for an interview. At eighty-two, Marvin's mother had been diagnosed with end-stage renal failure. "We thought Mom was perfectly healthy," Marvin said. "She went to see her doctor for what she thought was a bladder infection, and now they're telling us her kidneys are shutting down."

"Is dialysis an option?" I inquired.

"She's refusing it," he replied.

"Has she given you any indication of her end-of-life wishes?"

Abruptly, Marvin stood and placed his hand over his wife's stomach, visibly angry. "How can you discuss death with my pregnant wife in the room? It could be harmful to our baby." I was taken aback by his reaction. Marvin was a sophisticated entrepreneur, yet he believed that the mere mention of the word "death" could cause harm to his unborn child.

Whether we talk about it or not, death is a natural and certain phenomenon in our lives. Nonetheless, I have often seen people knock on wood when the word is mentioned, as though a superstitious gesture could ward off the unwelcome event. Others feel that death will just take care of itself and prefer not to discuss it. Unfortunately, leaving no plan adds only more grief and heartache to an already sorrowful event. Have your parents made their end-of-life decisions? Have they left directives for your family? By discussing and preparing for death, we lessen the mystery of it and give ourselves some control.

Everyone knows how they would like to die—quickly and without pain. Contrary to our hopes, death more often comes slowly and progressively due to technology that offers options not available a generation ago. Today more than ever, preparation for death is vital.

There is no easy way to rally people's enthusiasm for acknowledging and planning for death, but as those who have already experienced a death in the family know, death requires preparation. Bring up the subject before a medical crisis occurs. Once your parent becomes ill, it is harder to discuss.

Thelma. "I'll tell you what a good death would be," commented ninety-eight-year-old Thelma. She and her daughter Agnes and I had been discussing the death of Walter Matthau. "I want family around me, but not crying. I want to go quickly. No pain, please, and no tubes or needles of any kind. I'd hate to be a burden to my children, and my body will be tired anyway—it's had a pretty good run!" she laughed.

By being clear about how she envisioned her own death, Thelma was empowering her daughter for the future. Agnes would never have to decide whether to be aggressive about her mother's care. There would be no room for regret.

During the past thirty-seven years I have traveled through the dying process with thousands of families. I have witnessed peaceful, pain-free death. I have also witnessed death prolonged far longer than it should have been, with more suffering than necessary. Too often, I have seen families emotionally and financially drained because their parents left them no directives.

Megan. Megan, eighty-four, was admitted to our nursing home following a massive stroke, which left her unable to swallow. The question arose: Should a feeding tube be inserted into her stomach? Her two daughters found themselves confused and at odds. When Jeannie stated emphatically that she wanted no heroics, Monica countered, "I can't make that call. No one can. We need to put the tube in." Since Megan had left no plan, there were hard feelings between her daughters, both of whom were arguing for what they assumed their mother would want.

For families of frail, elderly parents, the question of whether or not to extend life can be agony. We must be clear about when to take advantage of technology and when not to. According to Robert Butler, founder of the National Institute on Aging, "Americans are only beginning to wrestle with the emotional issues of life support. That's a national conversation that's going to take twenty years."

Taking Control

Just as you want control over your life, you will want that same control over your death. Frightening as the topic is, much of the fear lies in avoidance. Talking about death and planning for it can give you a measure of control over your parent's death as well as your own. In fact, discussing end-of-life preferences with your parents is one of the most meaningful and compassionate conversations you can have. Since the majority of us do not wish to be kept alive by a tube or a machine, it is essential that your parent's wishes regarding end-of-life decisions be honored. Talking about the final journey as a family enables each of us to make appropriate decisions and increases the probability that a parent's directives will be carried out.

Everyone's death is as unique as his life. Those of us who have been fortunate enough to have one or both of our parents reach their eighties, nineties, or even one hundred realize that the downside of a long life is meeting the challenge of adult caregiving as their needs intensify and they become more frail. More than death itself, people fear a prolonged dying process. Given that death is inevitable, there may come a time when your focus on aggressive medical curing shifts to nonaggressive, compassionate caring.

How Do You Talk About Death?

"Only my daughter," laughed my father as we sat on a bench in the backyard, "asks me about dying on such a beautiful, sunny afternoon." I could sense that Dad was debating whether to proceed with the conversation. As my parents entered their mid-seventies, I knew they had made no preparations, nor had they talked to anyone in the family about their end-of-life wishes. That particular afternoon, the timing seemed right. I tried to keep the tone of the conversation unthreatening and focused on the fact that if Dad communicated his wishes now it would allow him to keep control in the future. The conversation with my father shed new light on the awkwardness of this emotionally loaded subject.

"Honey," Dad said, "I don't worry about what happens after I die. I do worry about what it will be like before I die." Many years passed, and our summer conversation became the first of several on this personal topic. At the time of each of my parents' deaths, I felt empowered to follow through on their directives. Each parent left clear, complete directions. Any uncertainty or anxiety I experienced was greatly reduced. I took comfort in knowing I had followed their wishes.

Should you find that your parent is not ready to discuss the topic, try again later. The right timing will increase the likelihood that your message will be heard. Rehearse your words and wait for the right opportunity; the subject may come up unexpectedly. Sensitive issues are better discussed in person, since it allows you to observe your parent's body language and facial expressions. If he is looking uncomfortable, you will be better able to decide if it is time to back off or to change your approach. Sometimes a light touch will let him know you are there for him. The manner in which you speak is as important as what you say.

The subject of death is a two-edged sword. On the one side, we contemplate our parent's death, and on the other, we face our own. During the question-and-answer period following a workshop I presented on death and dying, an eighty-six-year-old gentleman raised his hand and asked, "What if *I'm* ready and want to talk to my kids about my wishes and *they* can't deal with the subject?"

If your parent says, "You know, I'm not going to live forever," or "I hope I'm still here five years from now," he may be opening the door for some meaningful conversation. It is normal to want to reassure him by saying, "You've got lots of years left, Dad," or to laugh it off by joking, "Don't be silly, Dad, you're going to outlive us all!" But are you listening to what he is saying to you? If your parent is ready to discuss final wishes, and you cut the communication off, he may feel that you are unable to deal with his possible illness or death. He may move into "parent mode" to protect you from a disturbing conversation.

You may have to enter uncomfortable territory in order to talk about death with your parent. One way to keep this conversation going and hear more about your parent's wishes is to repeat the end of his sentence with a question. If you parent says, "You know I'm not going to live forever," you can answer, "Not going to live forever? Does that frighten you?" Don't miss this opportunity to allow your parent to share his feelings. Getting in touch with your own feelings on this topic will affect your ability to have a meaningful discussion.

Letting Go

"Mom just won't let go," cried Tina, visibly shaken as she walked into my office. "How can anyone so weak continue to live? She hasn't had anything to drink or eat for five days. The thought of losing her is overwhelming, but Mom is worn out and—as heartless as it may sound—she needs to slip away."

I have witnessed families who prayed that their parent's death would take place sooner rather than later. Then, in the next breath, they accuse themselves of being unloving. "Tina," I said, "holding on to your parents is a basic human instinct. However, holding on is no longer as important as letting go."

There are times when a resident's dying process goes on longer than usual. Remind your parent how much she is loved, and how important she has been to you and your family. Tell her something like, "I'm okay, Mom. My children are okay. You have taught us well. When you are ready, complete your journey in peace." Have other family members give similar affirmations and reassurances. My experiences with families are by no means a scientific study, but I have often seen that giving people permission to die can be an invaluable final gift. You will find that the peace you share with your parent will bring you peace as well.

Charlotte. "How could this happen?" said Charlotte, crying in her mother's room. "I was by Mom's side for twelve straight hours. I left for thirty minutes to get a hamburger and she died while I was gone. It's not fair."

Her experience is not uncommon. "Charlotte," I replied, "I have seen residents die when a family member leaves the room for a short time; I have seen others wait until a certain family member arrives. Our parents will travel through death in their own way, in their own time. There was a reason for your not being with your mother at the final moment. She may have continued to mother you and protect you as long as you were sitting there. Once you left, she was able to slip away."

How we anticipate our parents' death—with acceptance or with dread—will depend on how much we have prepared for it. Only they can tell us how they want their final days managed. No one can predict the future, nor can we guarantee it will be trouble-free. But you can help make your parents' final journey a positive experience. Their deaths will always remain in your memory. Work together to make it a peaceful one.

❝Help!" cried Harriet as she walked into my office. "I just found out Mom didn't pay her Medigap premium for six months. She had out-patient cataract surgery and now I'm getting billed for hundreds of dollars that Medicare didn't cover. When I reapply for Medigap, it's going to be more expensive because of her age and preexisting illness. She may even be denied coverage altogether!" Harriet continued, "A friend told me if I enroll Mom in an HMO, it will be cheaper and less hassle. I didn't even know I *could* change Medicare to an HMO. What should I do?"

"Harriet," I sighed, "welcome to the 'Medi' world. Medicare, Medigap, Medicare Advantage, and Medicaid are terms you need to be familiar with for your mother's benefit as well as your own."

As our society ages, each program becomes more complex. Regulations, varying from state to state, are constantly being revised and amended. Although the Internet can be helpful, sorting through the maze of information can leave you frustrated and paralyzed. I have assembled broad definitions of the basic plans, but be aware that an attorney in your state who specializes in estate planning or elder law can give you the best advice.

MEDICARE

In 1965, Medicare became the federal government's principal insurance health-care program to cover basic needs for people sixty-five years of age and older (and for certain disabled people under sixty-five). Almost all Americans sixty-five or over who have paid into the Social Security system receive Medicare as their basic health-care insurance program. Those who worked a minimum of ten years of Medicare-covered employment during their lifetime (or were married to a spouse who did) are eligible.

The Social Security Administration, which oversees the eligibility and enrollment process, recommends applying for Social Security benefits ninety days prior to the day you wish to begin receiving payments. Your parent may choose to apply as early as age sixty-two, but he will not receive the full amount he would have received if he had waited until he was sixty-five. From age sixty-five to seventy, your parent can slightly increase his benefits for every month he waits. Regardless of when he chooses to begin receiving Social Security, he must apply for Medicare at age sixty-five. (If he applies for Social Security at sixty-five, he will automatically receive his Medicare card.) If he chooses to start receiving Social Security at an older age, he must still apply for Medicare at the Social Security office between three months before and three months after his sixty-fifth birthday. Should he miss this specific enrollment period, he will face penalties and delays. To find out which government benefits your parent is eligible for, visit www.benefitscheckup.org or contact your local Social Security office.

The A, B, Cs, and Ds of Medicare. Medicare is currently divided into four parts, and will probably be divided further as time goes on. Traditional Medicare (Parts A and B) and Medicare Part D are available throughout the United States. Medicare Advantage, Part C, may be an option depending on where you live and what plans are available in your community.

Part A—The Hospital Insurance

Medicare Part A covers medical and psychiatric inpatient hospital expenses, a limited number of days for skilled nursing following a hospital stay, and hospice care. Following a hospitalization, it may also cover home health care for a period of time. If your parent is entitled to Social Security benefits, he is eligible for Part A free of charge—there are no premiums for this part of Medicare; however, there is a yearly deductible that will increase annually. If your parent is over sixty-five, and is not eligible for Medicare, he may still be able to participate as a "voluntary enrollee" by paying monthly premiums as long as he is a U.S. citizen or a legal resident for five years.

Part B—The Medical Insurance

Medicare Part B helps cover outpatient services such as doctor bills and outpatient hospital services, as well as physical and occupational therapy and other health services. It also covers diagnostic tests, durable equipment, and ambulance transportation. In 2005, Medicare Part B began to cover some preventative procedures, including a one-time initial physical exam within six months of enrollment in Part B. It also covers screening for early detection of heart disease and diabetes, as well as flu shots, pneumonia vaccine, Pap smears, mammography, and bone mass measurement. It does not cover nursing home care.

If your parent is eligible for Part A, he will automatically be enrolled in Part B. While your parent can opt not to enroll in Part B, he would then be financially responsible for all nonhospital medical bills. Part B enrollees pay a monthly premium that is automatically deducted from their Social Security checks. In 2006, the Part B premium deducted from Social Security was increased to $88.50. Beginning in 2007, high-income beneficiaries will pay more for their Medicare Part B premiums, based on a sliding fee scale—the higher your income over $80,000, the higher your premium. Your parent must meet an annual deductible for Medicare Part B, at which point Part B will pay 80 percent of what Medicare considers a "reasonable charge," and your parent will be responsible for the remaining 20 percent coinsurance. (Coinsurance is a percentage of the costs per service, as opposed to copayment, which is a flat fee for each service.)

If your parent decides to enroll in Part B at a later date, he will pay a higher monthly premium. For each year he does not enroll in Part B, his monthly premium will increase by a permanent 10 percent; if your parent waits four years to enroll in Part B, his monthly premium will be permanently 40 percent higher than it would have been initially. (This penalty does not apply if he is still working and currently covered by an employer group, former employer, or a retirement plan.) Like Part A, Medicare Part B has specific enrollment periods for those who elect to enroll at a later date. General enrollment is January 1 through March 31, with coverage becoming effective in July. If your parent initially decides not to take Part B, he will have to wait for the next enrollment period. If he is still working, he is entitled to a special eight-month enrollment period after he retires or after he loses his employer-sponsored health insurance.

As the government tries to contain health-care costs, Medicare deductibles, premiums, and coverage are in a constant state of flux. The most dependable way to obtain current information is to call 800-633-4337. (These numbers spell out the word Medicare.) Or go to www.medicare.gov.

Medigap. Medigap is a supplementary or secondary health insurance policy sold by private companies to fill in the "20 percent gap" that traditional Medicare Part B does not cover. Although the plans are designed to pay the coinsurance and deductibles associated with payment for hospital care services, you must be aware that Medigap will not cover any service not covered by Medicare; it is strictly a supplement to Medicare coverage. With all the premiums, deductibles and coinsurances that exceed Medicare-approved charges, *supplemental insurance is crucial.* Your parent should apply for a policy at the same time he receives his Medicare Part B insurance. As long as he applies within six months of enrolling in Medicare Part B, a Medicare recipient cannot be denied a Medigap policy or be charged more due to preexisting conditions. If your parent misses this six-month period, the insurance company can increase the price of the policy, ask your parent to sign a preexisting condition clause of exclusions, or refuse coverage altogether due to a preexisting condition. (For further information, call your state or city Health Insurance Counseling and Advocacy Program [HICAP]. Volunteer counselors are available to give free assistance with Medicare enrollment and entitlement, as well as Medigap and premium issues.)

Insurance companies offer ten standard Medigap packages, ranging from the basic Plan A to the most comprehensive Plan J.

Because premiums vary between insurance companies and from state to state, you must be careful when choosing one. Some states do not offer all the plans—instead, they offer policies similar to managed care, known as Medicare SELECT. With Medicare SELECT, patients are required to use a designated group of doctors, clinics, and hospitals.

Medigap does not cover long-term custodial care, unlimited prescriptions, vision care, dental care, hearing aids, or informal help at home. Premium prices are likely to increase annually. If your parent moves to another state in which his current insurance company is not available, he will have sixty days to purchase a Medigap policy. Go to www.Medicare.gov/MGCCompare to find the plans available in your parent's geographic area and to get tips on buying the right policy.

In an attempt to keep health-care costs under control, Medicare assigns a "reasonable charge" for a service or procedure. If Dr. Black "accepts assignment," he has agreed to accept this Medicare-approved payment as 80 percent of his fee with the remaining 20 percent paid by a Medigap policy. Without Medigap insurance, your parent will have to pay the 20 percent coinsurance.

If Dr. Green, also a Medicare-approved physician, does *not* accept assignment, he can charge as much as 15 percent over the Medicare-approved amount. After the Medicare and Medigap reimbursements are made, your parent will have to pay the remaining 15 percent of the bill.

Dr. White is not a Medicare-approved physician. A patient who chooses to see him will be responsible for 100 percent of the bill.

Always ask if your doctor accepts Medicare assignments. If you fail to ask, you may be in for a financial surprise. Before choosing any Medigap plan, read the fine print for preexisting condition exclusions. If your parent is thinking about joining an HMO, or if he is close to exhausting his funds and will soon be eligible for Medicaid, a Medigap policy is not needed.

Part C: Medicare Advantage Plans—an Alternative to Parts A and B

In the Balanced Budget Act of 1997, Congress created Medicare Part C in another attempt to keep Medicare financially sound. The idea was to increase the number of seniors receiving health care from managed-care plans rather than from traditional Medicare. Your parent can stay in the original Medicare or opt to disenroll, and enroll in one of the available Part C Medicare Advantage Plans. Each of these plans provides a different type of coverage, and some plans may not be offered in all areas. Since there are significant variations among Medicare Advantage plans, read through all the information from government and nonprofit sources. Being an informed consumer is the best way to make the right Medicare choices. You can find up-to-date information at Medicare's website. Go to www.medicare.gov/MPPF for the "Medicare Personal Plan Finder." If your parent does not choose a particular Part C plan, he will automatically be enrolled in traditional Medicare.

Part C Medicare Advantage Plans include

Health Maintenance Organization (HMO)
and HMO with Point of Service Plan (POS),
Preferred Provider Organizations (PPO),
Private Fee for Service (PFFS), and
Medicare Specialty Plan

When your parent joins a Medicare Advantage Plan program, he is still part of Medicare, but he is agreeing to receive benefits from his managed-care provider. The Medicare Advantage Plan will probably be less expensive, require minimal deductibles, and offer your parent benefits not covered under traditional Medicare such as prescription, dental, and vision care. Additionally, all Part C plans eliminate the need for a Medigap policy. To qualify for any of these plans, your parent must be receiving both Medicare Parts A and B. Your parent will continue to have the premium for Part B deducted from his Social Security check.

The HMO. In 1986, HMOs were presented to the sixty-five-and-older demographic as a comprehensive answer to traditional Medicare, which had burdened recipients with deductibles, coinsurance, Medigap insurance premiums, and unending paperwork. HMOs are the least expensive, but the most restrictive of the Part C Medicare Advantage Plans. HMOs hold out the tantalizing promise of no Medicare deductibles or coinsurance charges, thus eliminating the need for Medigap insurance. As usual, when something sounds too good to be true, it probably is. The government's goal for managed care was to place a limit on unnecessary tests and procedures, but in my experience, managed-care patients receive fewer needed health services than traditional Medicare patients, making constant family involvement critical if your parent is to receive essential medical attention. HMOs widen their profit margin by doing less for the elderly. Learn your parent's rights because at some point you may need to take charge of his health care. *By law, the HMO plans must offer everything traditional Medicare offers.* The challenge is obtaining the coverage.

Under HMO coverage, only your parent's primary physician can refer your parent to a specialist, and that specialist must be an

HMO provider. Thus, the HMO physician is the "gatekeeper" to further care. Receiving this doctor's permission is not always easy. Many HMO primary care physicians attempt to care for all their patients' medical problems themselves with little reliance on specialists, who are only recommended if urgently necessary or if the family demands it.

Managed-care plans keep costs down by limiting a patient's doctors, hospitals, and nursing homes to a list of network providers. Medicare pays a set amount of money each month for each patient in the plan, and the HMO keeps whatever is not spent on health care. As your parent ages and needs more health care, he may be viewed as a financial liability and may not receive the diagnostic tests he needs. Be vocal if you are not satisfied with your parent's care. Ask for the customer relations department of the HMO, or use the Internet to contact your state or city Health Insurance Counseling and Advocacy Program office. If your parent chooses to see a provider outside the HMO network, he will have total financial responsibility for his choice—Medicare will not pay for his visit.

If your parent finds that the HMO is not working for him, he can return to traditional Medicare by requesting a disenrollment form from the managed-care plan, by calling Medicare at 800-633-4337, or by visiting a Social Security office. Until 2006, it was fairly easy to leave a managed-care plan and return to traditional Medicare; but starting in 2006, there is a "lock-in" period—beneficiaries can change plans only once a year during a six-month period, which will be shortened to three months in coming years.

The catch to reentering traditional Medicare is that your parent will need supplementary insurance. Since Medigap insurance companies have the right to refuse your parent or charge him a higher rate due to preexisting conditions, your parent may have to continue with the HMO. Check his membership contract for details about any denied coverage you feel he is entitled to. The contract will specify a process for appeals that must be followed to gain the care he needs.

The HMO with Point of Service Plan (POS) is a combination of the HMO and the PPO health insurance plans. It is a more attractive plan, but it is also more expensive. Like an HMO, the POS assigns your parent a primary care physician. The difference is that the POS allows your parent to use doctors and hospitals outside the POS-approved provider network as long as the primary physician refers him. Getting a referral for a specialist may prove difficult. If a member does see a non-network physician, the POS plan pays a portion of the cost and the member picks up any additional charges. If your parent can afford out-of-pocket expenses, he gains access to more physicians, particularly specialists. Keep in mind costs can add up if your parent regularly uses out-of-network physicians.

Preferred Provider Organization (PPO). A Preferred Provider Organization is a combination fee-for-service/managed-care plan. PPOs are networks of primary care physicians, hospitals, and support services that provide medical service to specific groups or associations. If your parent chooses this plan, he retains more choice over physician and hospital care than with the HMO plans. Although he is allowed to choose health providers outside the network, he will face a higher coinsurance. PPO patients do not usually need a referral to see specialists, but check the policy! They may need to go through the primary care physician. There may also be a monthly premium. As with all Part C choices, PPOs eliminate the need for Medigap. PPOs may offer additional benefits, such as annual physicals, preventative services, and prescription drug benefits. Before using any out-of-network doctor, your parent must ask if he accepts the PPO's partial payment. If he does not, your parent will be responsible for all charges.

Private Fee-for-Service (PFFS). The PFFS is a Medicare-approved private insurance plan. It will include all Medicare Part A and B benefits while providing additional benefits at further cost. Like the original Medicare, your parent may go to any doctor or hospital that agrees to provide care under the PFFS terms and conditions. The private insurance company sets the amount of money it will pay and how much your parent will be required to pay for a service. Like traditional Medicare, the health-care provider is allowed to bill your parent up to 15 percent more than the PFFS-allowed charge, and your parent will have to pay the difference. While this plan provides unlimited choice of providers, total cost to PFFS members is likely to be higher than traditional Medicare program fees due to unlimited premiums and higher out-of-pocket costs. This plan may not be available in all parts of the country. Again, go to www.medicare.gov/MPPF for more information.

Medicare Specialty Plans. Medicare is working to create specialty plans, which are new ways to provide more focused health care for certain people. If available in your area, these plans are designed to supply all the usual Medicare health care as well as more focused care to manage specific diseases or conditions such as congestive heart failure, diabetes, or end-stage renal failure.

Part D—The Prescription Drug Benefit

With the passage of the Medicare Prescription Drug Improvement and Modernization Act of 2003 came a new prescription drug benefit called Medicare Part D, effective January 2006. After paying out-of-pocket the first $250 worth of prescriptions (the deductible), your parents are responsible for only 25 percent of the next $2,000 (that is, $500). At this point, Medicare coverage actually stops and your parents are responsible for 100 percent of the next $2,850 themselves. This $2,850 for which your parents have no coverage is called the coverage gap, or "doughnut hole."

$250 the deductible
$500 25 percent of the next $2,000
+ $2,850 the "doughnut hole"
_____
$3,600 out-of-pocket expenses

When total out-of-pocket drug expenditures reach $3,600, Medicare drug coverage starts again. From then on, your parents will qualify for "catastrophic benefits" and for the remainder of the year, they will only pay $2–$5 copayments or 5 percent of the drug cost, whichever is greater.

A further cost is the premium: an estimated $35/month ($420/year) in 2006. Enrollment is not automatic, but rather voluntary. If seniors do not enroll in Part D in the first six months they are eligible, and then later decide to join, they will have to pay higher premiums—a penalty of about 1 percent of the premium for each month they delay. Each year, deductibles and your parents' out-of-pocket costs start all over again and, of course, each year the deductible, the copayments, and premiums will increase based on overall Medicare drug spending. The initial enrollment period will run from November 15 to December 31 of the year prior to the year for which your parents are enrolling. At any time during the first three months of the year, your parents will be able to change their prescription drug plan; after that, they are locked in.

Under the new law, low-income seniors receive special help, although there is a strict assets test that may disqualify some from receiving assistance. There are multiple levels of low-income aid, and each state has its own eligibility qualifications. Impoverished individuals may not have to pay monthly premiums and deductibles, and may be protected from the "doughnut hole." For low-income residents in nursing homes, copayments are waived.

Medicaid (Medi-Cal in California and Mass Health in Massachusetts)

Created in 1965, Medicaid is a health insurance program administered by each state jointly with the federal government for people living at or below poverty level. Every state determines its own eligibility requirements and oversees its own Medicaid program. Being eligible for Medicare does not necessarily mean you are eligible for Medicaid; your parents must verify that their income and assets do not exceed the amount set by their state of residence. If your parents qualify, they will not need additional Medigap insurance.

Medicaid, the nation's largest payer for nursing home care, covers many expenses that Medicare does not. It helps seniors with prescription drug costs as well as hearing aids and dental care. It also pays the Medicare deductibles, all coinsurance, and the monthly Part B premium. In short, whatever Medicare does not pay for, Medicaid will cover. Since Medicaid limits what the medical industry can charge, it is not surprising that a significant number of physicians and nursing homes are withdrawing from the program or limiting the Medicaid patients they will care for.

Your parents can apply for Medicaid at your county welfare office, public health department, or state social service agency. Because each state is continually reworking the eligibility requirements and restrictions, check with the local welfare office for the most current guidelines and procedures. For the most up-to-date, state-appropriate information, call Eldercare Locator at 800-677-1116 to request the

217

phone number for your local Area Agency on Aging, or go to www .n4a.org. You can also contact the Centers for Medicare and Medicaid Services (CMS) at www.cms.hhs/gov.

Joanna and Chuck. Joanna, eighty-seven, called me at my office one afternoon asking if I accepted Medicaid patients. "My husband and I taught our kids to save their money and make good business decisions. When my son recommended that we transfer our assets into his name, it seemed to make sense. That way if we ever needed nursing home care, the state would pick up the tab. So we did it. Well, now my husband Chuck is in a nursing home, and the care he is receiving is barely adequate. My friends tell me it's because most of the patients in the home are on Medicaid—welfare. Every time I go see him, it breaks my heart. We had no idea how limited the care would be on Medicaid. I told my son I may need our money back if Medicaid can't provide the care I want for Chuck."

The advantage of paying privately for nursing home care is that your parents are more likely to gain entrance to the facility of their choice because they will be paying a higher daily rate than Medicaid recipients. Families whose parent is close to exhausting his funds should relocate him to a combination private pay/Medicaid facility as a private paying resident. Then, when your parent exhausts his funds, the nursing home must allow him to stay. The facility's social worker can help fill out the tedious Medicaid application. Should your parent exhaust his funds in a facility that does *not* accept Medicaid reimbursement, the social worker can give you the names of facilities in the area that do have Medicaid contracts. Generally, the better the mix of private-paying patients, Medicaid patients, and Medicare (rehab) patients, the better the chance that it is a facility offering an adequate level of care.

Medicaid Planning. For married couples, long-term care can cause financial ruin and loss of the family home. "Medicaid planning" is a legal way of rearranging finances in order to make one spouse eligible for the Medicaid program without impoverishing the other. In 1988, the Medicare Catastrophic Coverage Act (also known as the Spousal Impoverishment Protection Law) became federal law and allowed a couple's assets and income to be divided so that a spouse will not lose everything should his partner need nursing home care. If your parents' assets have not been handled properly, their Medicaid nursing home coverage may be in jeopardy and both spouses may lose assets they are entitled to keep. Rules vary from state to state, but all Medicaid programs require complicated income and asset limits. Even if you feel your situation is straightforward, it is critical to seek the advice of an elder-law attorney who is familiar with the Medicaid process in your parent's home state. Do this before attempting to qualify for coverage.

"Spending down" is the term for using up savings in order to meet Medicaid eligibility requirements. Your parent cannot apply for Medicaid until he spends down his savings to whatever the state law considers poverty level. Currently in California, an individual has to spend down to $2,000; for a couple, it is $3,000. Many states are currently revising and tightening financial eligibility requirements, and the recent trend has been to extend Medicaid "look back" periods for investigating an applicant's true financial condition. In other words, the government will be looking for excessive spending down or gift giving, which is solely for the purpose of hiding assets and applying for welfare.

As a society, are we choosing not to spend our savings on our own end-of-life care? Should the creative financial planning of seniors become the financial burden of other taxpayers? The discussion of Medicaid planning as a means of sheltering parents' assets provokes strong emotional response; opinions differ as to whether it is legal, ethical, or even advantageous. This issue will not be resolved here, but after years of working in nursing homes that contract with Medicaid, I recommend that families think twice before transferring funds out of their parent's name to qualify for Medicaid. Medicaid pays only for "minimum care," which often translates to substandard care. When the majority of residents are on Medicaid, reimbursement is so low that the nursing home is forced to operate understaffed. Additionally, with Medicaid there is no flexibility in long-term-care options—it only covers nursing homes. If your parent transfers his assets and then needs assisted-living care, Medicaid will not pay for this level of care. Your parent may find himself with no available funds for his care, unless he enters a nursing home—which he may not need. In other words, he may have traded valuable assets for minimum health care.

Quality Medicaid facilities do exist, but you need to do your homework to find them. (See Chapters 12 and 14 for how to choose a nursing home.) If your parent lives in an area where Medicaid facilities are the only option, I highly recommend that your family become actively involved and ask the nursing staff what you can do to help care for your parent. You will find family participation produces a higher level of care from the facility.

LONG-TERM-CARE INSURANCE

In her late sixties, Sue bought long-term-care insurance. "I had a feeling I'd need help," she said, "and I didn't want my girls worrying about me and I didn't want government aid." Now eighty-four, Sue is an assisted-living resident and her long-term-care policy is providing $100 a day toward her care for three years. Although her room rate is $4,000 per month, between her Social Security, a small pension, and the long-term-care benefit, she will not have to delve into her savings for three years. For Sue, long-term-care insurance paid off.

Traditionally, families have paid privately (out-of-pocket) for home care and assisted living. For nursing home care, they relied on either private funds or Medicaid. Now, long-term-care insurance offers a third alternative.

While most insurance provides coverage for the unexpected, this insurance covers the expected—barring an early death, we will all assuredly grow old and need assistance. With most types of insurance, the insured hopes never to use the coverage. With long-term-care insurance, the majority of insured will need the benefits.

A quality long-term-care insurance policy will cover expenses that Medicare will not; for example, home health care, adult day care, assisted living, or a skilled-nursing facility. It can increase your chance of remaining financially independent and staying home as long as possible. Long-term-care insurance will help you to live where you choose, receive the kind of care you need, and determine who will deliver that care.

Who is a candidate for long-term-care insurance? There are no guidelines that cover everyone, and there are as many reasons not to buy this insurance as there are to buy it. If your parent is eighty years of age or older, or suffers from a chronic progressive disease, this type of insurance is probably not an option. The cost would be so high that it would outweigh the value of the policy. Further, the insured must be able to commit to paying the premium (including unexpected increases) until he needs the benefit. Long-term-care insurance is not for someone whose funds will shortly run out, as he will soon qualify for Medicaid. Since the wealthy can afford long-term care and the poor will be taken care of by the state welfare program, it is middle America that needs to explore long-term-care insurance. Insurance companies recommend policies for those in their late forties and early fifties. However, this group already has competing financial priorities—children's education, mortgages, and retirement savings. A long-term-care insurance policy should not affect your standard of living.

That said, for someone in their late fifties to early seventies, long-term-care insurance may be worth looking into. More complicated than other types of insurance, these policies vary widely regarding what they cover, how much they cover, and how long coverage will last. Cost depends on age, health status, and type of benefits chosen. The long-term-care insurance industry is still in its infancy, and we are just beginning to see how effective it will be.

When you apply for a policy, you will be asked to decide: (1) a daily benefit amount, (2) the number of years you want the company to pay you this benefit, and (3) the deductible (the number of days or months before the company will begin paying after you qualify). Your premium will be based on these decisions as well as your age and current health status.

To begin receiving benefits, generally a policy holder must require assistance with two or more activities of daily living (ADLs). ADLs include bathing, dressing, eating, transferring from a bed to a chair, using a toilet, and managing incontinence. The patient's ability to accomplish these tasks is assessed by a licensed nurse who is an employee of the insurance company. In some cases, insurance companies require a doctor to certify that his patient requires assistance with ADLs.

Select your insurance agent carefully. Since you will be trusting him with your financial information and your long-term-care objectives, consider a good recommendation from a friend, accountant, or elder-law attorney. Approach the final decision with caution. Be aware that policies are loaded with contingencies that may keep you from receiving your benefits. Research, compare, and read the fine print. Since there are no standardized benefits, be sure your agent represents a number of insurance carriers so you have a variety of policies from which to choose. An experienced agent will help you determine whether you can afford this type of coverage and whether the policy you are considering will meet your needs in the future.

Two major concerns are whether the insurance company will be able to fund the flood of claims in the next twenty to thirty years, and whether the company will even be around that long. Should your insurance company fold, you could lose your coverage or face hefty increases by the company that buys it out. So choose a well-known company with assets in the billions that can withstand the financial onslaught of future claims. Before signing, have your agent review your rights should the company fail.

If an insurance company guarantees coverage by the following day, be wary. If they are not evaluating your health condition, they are probably not evaluating other applicants', either; you may end up in an insurance pool in which many people have preexisting conditions. In that case, either your premium increases will be significant or the company may default altogether.

Alice's Dilemma. Alice's husband had been a resident in our facility for seven years. Following his death, Alice continued to faithfully volunteer, helping residents during art classes. Now eighty, Alice huffed into my office one afternoon with a large folder full of insurance correspondence. "My long-term-care insurance premium has gone up again," she said, nearly hyperventilating. "I don't know what to do. I'm living on a fixed income and this is the second increase in thirteen years." Waving her policy in the air, she exclaimed, "This says I can stay at my current premium level only if I cut back on my benefits. I'm all alone. How can I know for sure if the insurance company will actually pay up when the time comes? I'm not sure this insurance was a good buy after all. Do they have the right to keep doing this?" she asked.

Yes. They do. The insurance company cannot raise just one person's premium, but it can petition the state's insurance regulators and prove that policy holders in a given pool of insured are costing more than the company can fund—in other words, that they are receiving more claims than they had estimated. Even if the company invests in stocks that drop in value, it may need to increase premiums to pay current claims.

Long-term-care insurance has been popular for only about fifteen years. Insurance companies are just beginning to see claims submitted by the first group of policyholders. As future costs become apparent, will you be able to meet the higher premiums on a fixed income? Or will continued increases render your policy unaffordable just at the time you need it?

Alice found herself in an unsettling situation. She could either increase her premium, reduce the length of her coverage, or increase her deductible. She could also walk away from the policy. On her monthly income, she could not afford the new premium. Deciding to scale back her benefit to keep the current premium, Alice cut the length of her coverage from four years to three. "At this rate, will I have any coverage at all by the time I need it?" she asked apprehensively. I couldn't answer her.

According to a *Consumer Reports* investigation, long-term-care insurance for most people is "too risky and too expensive." The investigators reviewed plans offered in California with regard to the safety of the financial institutions that offered them. Only three out of forty-seven measured up. The investigation revealed that the small print in many policies can keep you from collecting, and confirmed that there is no guarantee that these insurers will still be around two or three decades from now when you need them to pay.

The following definitions of long-term-care terminology may help you make a more informed purchasing decision.

Benefit Period. This is the length of time a policy will pay benefits, that is, how long you will receive financial assistance, designated in years from one year to life.

Daily Benefit. This is the maximum per-day amount a policy will pay for long-term-care services. Check out the cost of care in your area and do the math to determine the coverage you need. If you don't use the full amount of your daily rate, the unused portion remains in the value of your policy.

Elimination Period. The elimination period (also known as a deductible or waiting period), is the number of days you pay out-of-pocket before a policy's coverage begins. This period can range from zero to any number of days you select at the time you purchase the policy. The shorter the elimination period, the more expensive the policy will be.

Inflation Protection. An automatic inflation protection provision in the policy adjusts benefits to keep pace with inflation without increasing the premium. Without this protection, a policy can become virtually useless.

Preexisting Condition. This term refers to a condition or symptom for which medical advice or treatment has been given prior to applying for the insurance policy. When filling out the enrollment form, be as honest and accurate as possible. If you fail to mention an illness, the insurer may later decline to pay for a treatment related to the omitted condition, and may even terminate your contract.

Premium Waiver. With a premium waiver, once you qualify to receive benefits, you will no longer have to pay monthly premiums. However, since some policies do not provide premium waivers, you must check the small print.

Rated Policy. If you have a preexisting condition (such as diabetes or hypertension) that has future health-care risks to you and financial risks to the insurance company, the insurer may offer you a rated policy, one that takes specific potential costs into consideration and will have a rate higher than a standard plan.

Step-Down Provision. As the cost of monthly premiums increases—and it will if you do not have inflation protection—this provision allows you to reduce your benefits to keep your premium down. Without the step-down provision, you must meet the additional cost of each new premium increase.

Third-Party Notice. If your parent forgets to pay his monthly premium, the long-term-care insurance company must notify a specified third party—usually a family member—before the policy is terminated. This notice can be invaluable since a family is often unaware when a parent is beginning to be forgetful. Be sure to request this benefit.

Underwriting. All long-term-care insurance policies require some medical screening, called underwriting, which evaluates your health before you buy a policy. The stricter the underwriter, the better the chances that the premiums will not increase as often, since your parent will be classed with a healthier group of people. Some companies are less strict than others, but remember, companies boasting they can underwrite overnight will receive more claims and will be required to raise premiums more frequently.

ADVANCE DIRECTIVES

"Mom would not want to live like this," Joseph argued with his older sister, Jean, as they sat in my office. "She always said, 'Don't keep me around if I don't know who I am anymore.' Well, Mom's ninety now, and she doesn't know who she is, where she is, or even who we are. Using an IV to keep her alive when she can't swallow anymore goes against everything she wanted."

"I don't agree with you, Joe," Jean responded, "I just can't watch her starve."

"Jean, this is not about you," Joseph countered. "It's about Mom. If we can't agree on this, the doctor will continue to feed Mom through a needle in her vein forever!"

As dramatic as this exchange sounds, it is not uncommon when families find themselves with no written guidance. Whether it is a lack of information, fear of dealing with the subject, or disagreeing on the best course of action, many families enter the last caregiving phase without a clear definition of the medical care the parent would have wanted.

In 1991, the Patient's Self-Determination Act became federal law and changed the face of caregiving for the dying. It was the first law requiring hospitals and nursing home facilities to give residents and families written information explaining the right to refuse or accept treatment should the resident become incapacitated. Now, more and more families are aware of the importance of advance directives, written instructions to direct health care in the event the parent loses the ability to make or communicate medical decisions for himself. Without an advance directive, a hospital staff is required to aggressively keep the patient alive, possibly prolonging his suffering. An advance directive would have taken the burden off Joe and Jean at a time when they were emotionally upset by their mother's critical condition. But since their mother had not put her wishes in writing, she had no voice in her own care.

The two most common advance directives are the living will and the durable power of attorney for health care (DPA). Both are legal documents permitting your parent to set forth in writing his wishes regarding health care. A living will focuses exclusively on the medical treatment your parent wishes to receive when facing a terminal illness. A DPA goes a step further by assigning a representative to carry out the parent's wishes and to make decisions in his interest. In some cases, the two directives are compiled into one document. The living will and DPA can protect your parent from receiving aggressive, invasive medical care he would not have chosen. They can also allow him to request aggressive treatment. Planning ahead protects the parent, gives direction to the family, and is invaluable to the decision maker.

Advance directives must be signed *before* they are needed. If your parent is reluctant to talk about end-of-life decisions, be persistent while he is still healthy. If a relative or friend had a recent medical setback, you might use this as an opening to ask your parent what treatment he would have chosen if he were in the same situation.

Although the terminology, statutes, and documentation vary from state to state, an advance directive written in one state should be valid in all fifty. Even if an advance directive is not officially recognized in certain states, it can still serve as a guide to family members and health-care professionals when a person is no longer able to communicate his own wishes.

Most states have printed forms that meet all their requirements. A good source for forms approved by your state is Aging with Dignity (www.agingwithdignity.org). Many office-supply stores carry the forms, and they can also be downloaded from the Internet. Although the forms are self-explanatory, you may be more comfortable having an attorney prepare these documents.

The Living Will

In a living will, your parent describes how much medical intervention he wants regarding life-sustaining or life-prolonging medical treatment should he be unable to communicate his wishes to his health-care providers. Living wills are often used to tell the doctor to provide only treatment that keeps the patient pain-free when death is imminent and when aggressive treatment serves no purpose. In this way, they help to avoid inappropriate hospitalization. With a living will, your parent maintains control even at the end of his life. While the patient is still able to make his own decisions, a living will can easily be revoked. If your parent does revoke it, all known copies must be destroyed and his doctor and health-care providers notified. This will avoid confusion when another document is drawn up.

Because a living will is activated only when the patient is terminally ill or permanently unconscious, it is a limited directive; it does not direct actions for many clinical situations which may arise. Unlike a durable power of attorney for health care (DPA), the living will does not provide a health-care agent. Of these two forms, the DPA will prove to be the more valuable. In many states, the living will language is included in the DPA.

Durable Power of Attorney for Health Care (DPA)

This document allows your parent to appoint a representative to ensure that specified medical decisions are carried out. Also known as a "health-care agent," "proxy," or "surrogate," this person has legal authority to make health-care decisions on behalf of the patient at the time he becomes incapacitated, or otherwise unable to make medical decisions. Have your parent review the DPA with his physician. As the surrogate decision maker, the health-care agent can routinely remind the doctor of the parent's wishes.

Your parent should choose a decision maker who shares his values and whom he trusts to carry out his wishes. The health-care agent must fully understand the wishes as stated in the directives. If your parent chooses you, ask yourself if you are emotionally up to the task. Can you follow through on your parent's wishes to the end even if it includes no heroics? Even with the last wishes written out in black and white, there is often a great deal of guilt and emotional turmoil in carrying out a parent's last request. You must remember that you are not making the decision; your parent is. The directives merely guide and remind you to keep faith with your parent's wishes. Unless your parent specifies a shorter period of time (for example, following a life-threatening surgery), the DPA is valid indefinitely. A DPA can be revoked (canceled) at any time. A newly drawn-up form overrides all earlier directives.

Since it does not focus solely on impending death, the DPA covers a wide range of possibilities. It applies to all medical decisions, not just life-sustaining decisions, although it can specify treatments your parent does or does not wish to allow, such as surgery or artificial nutrition and hydration. The health-care agent can arrange a skilled-nursing facility, consent to specific medical procedures, and designate which life-sustaining treatments should or should not be used. Advance directives reduce the chance of conflict within the health-care facility where many crucial decisions are made. Perhaps more important, they prevent conflict, control struggles, and end debate among family members.

Vince and Bernice. "If only Dad had let us help him," said Vince, shaking his head in frustration, "my sister and I wouldn't be in this fix." Vince had stopped by to thank the staff for the care they had given his father.

"Dad wouldn't give Bernice or me a financial power of attorney, so we were never involved in any of his business transactions," Vince continued. "He left no will, no trust, and no directives as to

231

what to do with his estate. He never wanted to talk about his money. We just found out that he had a safe deposit box that the bank has now sealed. Who knows what's in it? He didn't think he had a large estate, but by the time you add up his bank account, stocks, home, car, and life insurance, there'll be more money than he realized. I'm afraid half of it will go to the government. Meanwhile, Bernice and I have to use our own money to pay his bills until probate is settled. What a nightmare."

If dealing with your parent's emotional and health-care issues feels overwhelming, try adding financial matters to your already full plate. For many families, this is an awkward, time-consuming responsibility. The consequences of not being prepared can be devastating and costly. Facing probate court proceedings, payment of unnecessary taxes, and other unexpected financial complications left Vince and Bernice little time to deal with their emotional loss. Too late, Vince realized how much was at stake. He should have been more persistent in encouraging his father to appoint a family member or associate to step in following his death to handle financial matters.

Have your parents protected their assets? Have they left instructions regarding who can step in and make legal decisions for them? No family should be without estate planning, even if the estate is modest. Many times, the value of an estate has grown dramatically without the rest of the family being aware of it. Estate planning will distribute your parents' assets according to their directions and minimize tax liabilities at the time of their death. Unnecessary fees, delays, and taxes can be avoided. Such planning allows your parents to control their assets both during and after their lifetime.

Encourage your parents to discuss financial concerns that may arise in the event of their death, or physical or mental incapacitation.

If they have not already prepared a will, a financial power of attorney, and a revocable living trust, discuss the benefit of doing so. If you are unable to persuade your parents, you may have to recognize that it is their decision and that they have the right to say that your involvement is not an option.

Financial information is a private matter, and discussing it may make you and your parents uneasy. You may fear appearing too interested in your inheritance. Your parents may fear losing control of their finances or fear that someone is trying to take their money. They may also be afraid of hurting one sibling's feelings when appointing another to be in charge of assets. Assistance from an elder-law attorney may reduce family tension while providing advice and assurance.

Discussing end-of-life money matters is a challenge for the best communicator. Too often I've witnessed adult children wait until a health crisis occurred, and by then it was too late. Look for opportunities such as the preparation of your own financial planning. Ask your parent for advice; then ask him what plans he has made. Since pressure frequently causes resistance, it may take more than one conversation. Keeping your parent as involved as possible will give him a feeling of control. Some families invite their parents to attend an estate-planning seminar or attend a class themselves and then share the valuable information they learn. Remember the "I" technique, mentioned in Chapter 4. ("I worry I won't be able to help you or know what to do if something happens." Or "I'll be able to relax if I know what you want me to do.") The goal is to speak frankly with your parent about his financial plans.

Role-play the conversation in your mind. When a quiet, relaxed time presents itself, you will be ready. Listen carefully to what your parent is saying. You will not organize everything overnight, but you will have opened up the subject for discussion. If you feel you are not the person best suited to deal with your parent's financial matters, choose the family member who is.

It is not uncommon for adult children to have no idea where their parent's legal documents are kept. Ask before a crisis takes place. The following is a list of documents you should be able to locate:

> *Durable power of attorney for health (or advanced health care directive)*
>
> *Durable power of attorney for finances*
>
> *Social Security card*
>
> *Certificates of birth, marriage, divorce, and citizenship*
>
> *Medicare card*
>
> *Medigap insurance card*
>
> *Auto insurance*
>
> *Property insurance*
>
> *Long-term-care insurance*
>
> *Life insurance*
>
> *Names of banks where they have checking and savings accounts or loans*
>
> *Names, addresses, and phone numbers of doctors, lawyers, financial advisers, and insurance agents*
>
> *Safe deposit box information (list of contents)*
>
> *Safe combination*
>
> *Most recent will*
>
> *Trusts*
>
> *Real estate deeds and mortgages*
>
> *Credit card information*
>
> *Bond and stock certificates, credit unions, money markets, and IRA plans*
>
> *Mutual fund accounts*

Pension plans and annuities
Veteran's benefits
Funeral, burial, and memorial instructions

Planning ahead gives your parents control of their assets. It ensures their choices, protects finances from mismanagement, avoids crisis decision making, and, most of all, reduces sibling anxiety and misunderstanding.

Financial Durable Power of Attorney

A financial power of attorney is a legal document that gives a spouse, relative, or trusted friend the power to make financial decisions for your parent should he become incapacitated. This power comes with a duty to act in the best interest of your parent as his legal agent. It gives the appointed person access to bank accounts to pay bills, submit insurance claims, and perform other personal financial tasks. Without a designated agent, financial matters will come to a halt upon the advent of a serious illness, as Vince discovered when he had to pay his father's bills out of his own pocket for several months. If there is no designated agent, a family member may have to petition the court to be appointed guardian or conservator—a lengthy, costly, and cumbersome process. If no family member steps forward, the state may appoint a nonrelative as legal guardian to handle the person's financial affairs.

The Will

Regardless of the size of the estate, a will ensures that the deceased's assets are distributed according to his stated wishes. Your parent can be very specific, creating a list of how he wants personal belongings such as jewelry, furniture, and clothing to be distributed among family members. If carefully thought out, a will may save a family years of squabbling and bad feelings.

A will usually has to be filed with the court in a legal proceeding called probate. In probate, a judge rules on the validity of the will, orders the payment of debts and taxes, and approves the distribution of assets. Without a will, your parent cannot select the beneficiaries of his own estate. Instead, the state will become the decision maker. Using a formula determined by state law, a court-appointed administrator will distribute the assets to beneficiaries. You may or may not agree with whom they appoint or with the administrator's decision regarding the distribution of assets. Charges for the administrator's services will be deducted from the estate. Further, your parent's assets may be on hold for many months, possibly years. Since the laws governing wills vary from state to state, it is always advisable to consult either an elder-law attorney or an attorney who specializes in estate planning.

Revocable Living Trusts

A living trust is a legal arrangement drafted by an attorney used in estate planning to provide a private and prompt distribution of assets to the beneficiaries without the need for probate court. Wealthy individuals use specially drafted living trusts to minimize estate and inheritance taxes. However, even for a modest estate, a living trust offers many advantages. A trust, unlike a will, requires no probate proceedings upon a person's death to transfer property to children, heirs, or beneficiaries. A trust has the advantage of being private and confidential, whereas a probate review of a will is a court matter open to the public. A living trust also has the advantage of allowing your parent to name in advance someone to step in as successor trustee to manage their financial affairs in the event they become physically or mentally incapacitated. If your parent regains his health or competency, he can resume his role as trustee. A living trust is flexible in that it can be changed or revoked at any time before death. After death, however, the trust cannot be changed. The successor trustee must follow your parent's wishes as stated in the trust document.

A living trust is much like running a family business. Your parent creates a trust into which he, as "trustor," transfers to another person, the "trustee," designated assets to manage. The trustee holds the property for the benefit of a third person—the "beneficiary." During his lifetime, your parent may simultaneously serve as trustor, trustee, and beneficiary while he continues to manage and control the trust property. In other words, while he is able, your parent creates, manages, and receives the benefits of the trust. If he dies or becomes incapacitated, a "successor trustee" named in the trust assumes the trustee position and follows instructions as stated in the trust. A revocable living trust estate plan will initially be more expensive than just a will, but it will save considerable legal fees in the future. As usual, the laws governing these legal proceedings vary from state to state. A revocable living trust must be prepared with the help of an elder-law or estate-planning attorney.

Irrevocable Trusts

Irrevocable trusts involve sophisticated tax planning dealing with a great number of tax laws. A trust of this kind cannot be changed or destroyed once it is created. The trustor turns over his ownership and control of his property. This form of trust provides an advantage in that the assets are no longer part of the estate, which may protect the beneficiary from having to pay inheritance taxes. The drafting of this type of arrangement requires specialized knowledge and experience in tax law. Only after consulting an elder-law attorney or an attorney who specializes in estate planning can your parent decide if this legal document is right for him.

Financial planning is not something you or your parent can afford to put off until later. One of the biggest mistakes families make is to wait until there is a health crisis, and by then it is often too late. For example, your parent must be mentally competent at the time he signs the estate-planning documents or they will not be considered valid.

Elder law has become such a specialty, with each state having different laws, that it makes good sense to work with a specialist in elder-law financial planning. Proper financial and estate planning with qualified professionals not only protects family assets from mismanagement and exploitation by others, it also reduces emotional upheaval when a crisis occurs. The expense of planning, while not insignificant, is nothing compared to the cost of not planning.

EPILOGUE

As I walked in the door, my son Christopher handed me the phone. "It's Vista," he said. "Silvia sounds nervous. I think it's about Nana."

"Stella, something's happening with your mom," said Silvia, the director of nurses. "She was just about to sit down for dinner when she started shaking and then fainted. She's in a deep sleep right now, and we're giving her oxygen. Her vital signs are stable. The doctor wants to know if you want her to go to the hospital."

Time stopped. Should I send Mom to the hospital? My mother's life was in my hands. I tried to remember her words. "I want no heroics, Stella," she had said. "If you can't bring me back in a better condition, then don't do it." My mother had chosen to avoid unwanted medical treatment and allow nature to take its course. The progression of her disease gave me my answer. There would be no hospital.

"Wait for me," I told Silvia. "I'll be right down." In

my car on the way, I did some soul-searching. How many hundreds of times I had reminded families that keeping their parent free of pain and discomfort becomes the ultimate goal. In my mother's case, hospitalization would be invasive and meaningless. Still, a wide range of emotions assaulted me: fear of making the wrong decision, anger that I had run out of options for my mother, sorrow about the loss awaiting me, and unexpected relief that I would no longer have to worry about Mom night and day, anticipating her many needs and changing my plans whenever she needed me.

When I arrived, I found Mom sleeping peacefully. My husband was already there. My son, brother, and sister-in-law were on the way. I called my two sisters who lived out of state. I knew Mom's death was imminent.

The next morning, Mom awoke and spoke in unexpectedly clear, meaningful sentences to each of us. Her words were an unbelievable gift. As I leaned over to kiss her, she whispered in my ear, "Stella, take care of yourself." These were her last words to me.

The following day, Mom stopped eating and drinking. Though I recognized this as a natural part of the dying process, I was not sure how to feel. I desperately wanted to do something, but there was nothing to do. Two days later, Mom died peacefully, surrounded by a family who loved her. Her death saved her from the final devastation of Alzheimer's. Her journey in this life had ended.

When I think about my mother's death, I am overwhelmed with sadness and happiness so intermingled; it is difficult to separate one emotion from the other. Initially, the loss was unbearable. I thought, I have lost both of my parents. I'm no longer anyone's child. Yet I was grateful that Mom's suffering had come to a merciful end.

Following my father's death years earlier, the time when I should have been grieving for him was taken up by assuming the caregiver role for my mother. While she mourned for my father, I busied myself watching over her. But now, my responsibilities as caregiver had come to an end. What a perplexing feeling—to be discharged from the most challenging, anxiety-provoking, and honorable position of my life.

The loss of my mother left me feeling vulnerable, mortal, and unable to move forward with my life. Later that week, while sorting through some of her belongings, I found a quote written on a 3 × 5 index card in her handwriting: "That which angers you conquers you!!" As I reread the sentence I pondered the word "anger." It had been underlined twice. Mom, my first teacher and guide, was once again showing me the way. I realized my uneasy reaction to her death was in fact due to anger that there was nothing I could do about it and that life was never going to be the same. This anger prevented me from dealing with my grief.

We all respond in our own way and in our own time to a grief that only time can heal. The death of a parent is a life-altering event, the final destination of the caregiving journey. On whichever windy road or detour you find yourself as you travel on the caregiving journey, remember: You are needed, you are doing the right thing, you make a difference. Most of all, don't forget my mother's advice: "Take care of yourself."

REFERENCES

Chapter 2. Red Flags: Ten Signs to Watch for in Your Parents

Lewis, George. "Adverse Drug Reactions Plague Elderly." *NBC Nightly News*. Health Report. 21 January 2004, http://www.drugawareness.org/Archives/1stQtr_2002/ Adverse_drug_reactionspla.html

Chapter 7. "My Mother Doesn't Have Alzheimer's, But..."

Evans, D. A., H. H. Funkenstein, M. S. Albert, et al. Prevalence of Alzheimer's disease in a community population of older persons: Higher than previously reported. *JAMA* 262, no. 18 (1989): 2552–56.

Fillit, Howard M., M.D. Dr. Fillit's commentary: A multidisciplinary approach to treating the patient with Alzheimer's disease (March 2001).

LTC Briefs. (Almost) 100% accuracy for diagnosing Alzheimer's. *Caring for the Ages*. (July 2004): 45.

Chapter 9. Caregiver Burnout

Department of Social and Health Services. Fact Sheet: Informal/ Family Caregivers. 1 December 2004, http://www.aasa.dshs.wa.gov/ professional/factsheets/informal%20and%20family%20caregivers .pdf.

Gardner, Amanda. Dementia caregivers go from distress to relief. *HealthDay News.* 12 November 2003, http://www.hon.ch/News/HSN/ 516005.html.

George, L. K., and L. P. Gwyther. Caregiver well-being: A multidimensional examination of family caregivers of demented adults. *The Gerontologist* 26 no. 2 (1986): 253–60. As cited by A. E. Scharlach, B. F. Lowe, and E. L. Schneider. *Elder Care and the Work Force: Blueprint for Action.* (Lexington, MA: Lexington Books, 1991).

Wart, Paula J., Caregivers need care too. *HealthPlus.* 11 September 2004. http://vanderbiltowc.wellsource.com/dh/Content.asp?ID=1387.

Yoshikawa, Thomas T., Elizabeth L. Cobbs, and Kenneth Brummel. *Practical Ambulatory Patients,* 2nd ed. (Philadelphia: Mosby-Yearbook, 1998), p. 46.

Chapter 11. Levels of Long-Term Care

Abrams, W. B., M. H. Beers, R. N. Butler, et. al. *Merck Manual of Geriatrics,* 2nd ed. (Whitehouse Station, NJ: Merck and Company, 1995).

Kimper, P., and C. M Murtaugh. Lifetime use of nursing home care. *New England Journal of Medicine* 324 (1991): 595.

Morris, Virginia. *How to Care for Aging Parents* (New York: Workman Publishing, 1996), p. 212.

Chapter 19. When and How to Visit

Ridder, Hanne Mette. Singing in individual music therapy with elderly persons suffering from Dementia. March 2000, http://www.musictherapyworld.de/modules/archive/stuff/papers/ HanneMe.pdf.

Chapter 23. Medicare, Medigap, Medicaid—Sorting Through the Maze

Do you need long-term care insurance? November 2003, http://www
.consumerreports.org. See: personal finance, long-term care insurance.

INDEX